The Clinical Laboratory in Nursing Education

Books of Related Interest

de Tornyay: **Strategies for Teaching Nursing, Second Edition,** *1982,*
0–471–04523–3

The Clinical Laboratory in Nursing Education

Second Edition

MARY SUE INFANTE, R.N., Ed.D.

Professor of Nursing
University of Connecticut
Storrs, Connecticut

A WILEY MEDICAL PUBLICATION
JOHN WILEY & SONS
New York · Chichester · Brisbane · Toronto · Singapore

Library of Congress Cataloging in Publication Data:

Infante, Mary Sue, 1939–
    The clinical laboratory in nursing education.

    (A Wiley medical publication)
    Bibliography: p.
    Includes index.
    1. Nursing—Study and teaching.   2. Medicine, Clinical.
I. Title.   II. Series.   [DNLM: 1. Education, Nursing—
United States.   2. Laboratories. WY 18 I43c]
RT73.I5   1985   610.73'07'11   84-25744
ISBN 0-471-88782-X

Printed in the United States of America

10 9 8 7 6 5 4 3 2 1

Preface to the Second Edition

The past decade has seen a number of studies conducted by nurse educators on various facets of the subject of the clinical laboratory in nursing education. Graduate students have pursued long-identified problems through theses and dissertations. Faculty have tested new approaches to clinical teaching. Faculty and graduate students alike have sponsored and attended scores of conferences on the subject, thus making possible dialogue among large numbers of new and seasoned nurse educators.

The upsurge of interest in the subject of teaching and learning in the clinical laboratory has been gratifying. It has also been rewarding to have had so many opportunities to converse with nurse educators committed to improving the most important part of our educational programs. Both verbal and written communications attest to the measured success of their efforts. All agree that much remains to be done. Yet there is a fuller development of the use of the elements, as well as expanded consideration of related subjects. The expectations of the nurse educator have heightened, and the mechanisms utilized to conduct and enhance clinical teaching have likewise increased. In addition, the demands for nursing practice have both changed and expanded.

This book provides faculty and graduate students of nursing with a unique approach to analyzing the purpose and use of the clinical laboratory in nursing education. It describes preparatory activities leading to optimal, efficient use of the clinical settings, as well as teacher and practitioner behaviors that should lead to more efficient outcomes. The subject matter deals with the "heart" of any nursing program of study, but it presents the subject matter in a manner that requires serious analysis and decision making by nurse faculty regarding future use of the clinical laboratory. It presents both challenges and wide ranging potential solutions to problems faced by educators in times of budgetary constraints and increased demands for scholarship and practice.

This second edition is both updated and expanded. It includes additional chapters on related areas. A chapter on the use of college laboratory, including simulation, provides examples of ways to improve the preparation of students for the best use of the clinical laboratory. Additional chapters on the use of clinical preceptors, consideration of other groups of people involved in the process of clinical teaching, and evaluation methods of clinical performance consistent with the teaching strategies proposed address current interests.

The book includes a focus on an aspect of teaching in professional education that is central to the socialization of the students in the role of the nurse. It is a useful source of information to graduate students of nursing preparing for the faculty role as well as an ongoing handy reference after graduation, and it provides an analysis of the teaching–learning process in the clinical setting. Novice and seasoned teachers alike will be stimulated by the suggested approaches to clinical teaching. In-service educators might consider application of the same concepts to the development of orientation programs for new graduates and planning for on-going educational programs for staff nurses. Nursing service administrators can utilize the concepts to set practice expectations as well as to guide them in the periodic evaluation of nurses in their agencies.

Clinical teaching is an immensely popular and intriguing subject, not only to nurse educators but to all nurses. This text should guide them to re-shape traditional thinking and experiment with different strategies. This is particularly important during times of "tight budgets" in higher education. The text contains suggestions for more efficient and effective use of clinical settings as well as needed research studies.

While much has been accomplished, much remains to be accomplished. A careful consideration and testing of the ideas and challenges that follow has the potential of improving the quality of clinical teaching and, ultimately, improving the quality of nursing practice. The challenge is indeed great as we prepare practitioners of nursing for the twenty-first century.

Mary Sue Infante

Preface
to the First Edition

Throughout the past several years, nurse educators have made valiant efforts to improve the quality of nursing education. As faculty members have improved their own level of education and have increased their knowledge of curriculum and teaching, they have initiated changes in nursing curricula. Therefore, in many instances, nursing has earned recognition in the academic world.

Curriculum changes, however, largely have been concerned with the identification and arrangement of content and course sequence. New teaching strategies and learning activities have been examined for their usefulness in nursing education. Many of these activities have been successfully incorporated into curricula where appropriate. It seems that the vast majority of these changes have been concerned with classroom teaching.

The clinical laboratory, which admittedly is a vital part of any professional curriculum, has essentially remained the same in character. Little systematic appraisal of its use, its purpose, and its activities has been conducted by nurse educators. Even young faculty members, fresh from graduate programs, tend to take this aspect of their teaching very much for granted. They teach much as they were taught.

This book on the essential elements of the clinical laboratory and the implications for the use of these elements in nursing education is intended to cast a new perspective on this sphere of preparation for practice. The inclusion of new concepts of clinical teaching in graduate programs will prepare teachers of nursing to practice in a new fashion. New and exciting avenues of possibility in the use of the clinical laboratory will become apparent. It should revitalize the use of the clinical setting in nursing education. It should result in more meaningful learning activities for students of nursing and more satisfying teaching activities for the teachers of nursing. A more thoughtful and creative practitioner will emerge. It will also become apparent that graduate students, preparing to teach, should be enticed to study and to continue research into the subject.

If changes in the use of the clinical laboratory, suggested here, are adopted, I believe they will have the potential for vastly new and different curricula. The more efficient use of faculty time and energies in laboratory activities will result in more efficient use of the resources of society in this educational endeavor. The higher level of the suggested learning activities of the students in such programs, hopefully, will stimulate inquiring minds that will render a quality health service today, and be prepared to search for the answers to problems in the delivery of health care for tomorrow.

Mary Sue Infante

Contents

CHAPTER 1

The Laboratory as an Educational Process

Currently, nursing has both the opportunity and the responsibility to practice in an independent and ever increasing interdependent role in health care. Clients entrusted to the care of nurses require knowledgeable, astute assessments, decision making, and creative applications of the intellectual and psychomotor skills of the nursing process. Curative and preventive research has resulted in more people surviving illness and accident as well as more people developing immunity to disease that they might otherwise have encountered. More people require maintenance and rehabilitative care, and more require support in advancing years. In short, more people are living longer.[1]

Even death and dying is prolonged. Subsequently, more people require the sustenance of comfort and the insurance of dignity throughout the process of dying. The current state of the "art of nursing" is that it is desperately needed by society—to a greater extent than ever before. The role of the nurse is heavily invested in prevention and promotion of health, and the maintenance and rehabilitation of chronic and long-term disorders. There are also increasing demands on the nurse in acute care or crisis-oriented care, although such episodes are of shorter duration for each person and family, and are heavily dependent upon medical interventions.

These societal circumstances present challenge and opportunity to nurse educators. They present a stage for dramatizing the fullest potential of the nurse. At the same time, it becomes quite evident that some current educational practices of the past will not suffice. The expectation is that of producing knowledgeable, competent, sophisticated practitioners. The means to meet this expectation is to design clinical activities that produce competent, confident, and respected practitioners of nursing. Clinical laboratory activities must be of the type, in the numbers, and under the circumstances likely to shape this kind of professional.

The clinical laboratory has had an important place in the history of nursing education. Its purpose has been much debated and questioned throughout this century. That it is an important part of the total curriculum for the preparation of professional nurse practitioners is undisputed. Students and teachers alike have spent long and exhausting hours in this setting. It has proven to be extremely costly for students and extremely time consuming for both students and their teachers. And all of this has continued to date in varying degrees for the express purpose of students "learning to give quality nursing care."

It is quite likely that you, like myself, have often asked: "Is this the best way to teach and to learn nursing?" "Is it the only way?" "Is it the most efficient way?" "Why have we done it, and why do we continue to do it in this way?" These questions actually plagued me during my years of clinical teaching in a baccalaureate program. Literature in nursing education identified problems, reported experimental teaching situations in the clinical laboratory, and even posed solutions to some problems. Changes were proposed without any real basis for the change being evident.

Although the clinical laboratory is an important part of the curriculum for the preparation of practitioners of nursing, during the past few decades relatively little study has been done on the use of the clinical laboratory in nursing education. At the same time, nurse educators seem to have become more and more aware of the need for more attention to the impact of the clinical setting in nursing education. They express concern and interest in what can be done to make it a more effective learning environment for the student. These same questions are raised at faculty meetings, continuing education programs for nurse educators, and conferences on nursing education. A sincere interest in how to improve clinical teaching while fulfilling the increasing demands of all other aspects of the nurse educator's role is most evident. Some individual faculty attempts to approach clinical teaching based on educational theory are notable. Yet, for the most part, the clinical laboratory, the heart of any professional program of study, is still used in essentially the same manner in all types of programs of study in nursing. Although the concern is there, and most nurse educators work diligently to alter curricula in an admirable fashion toward a theoretical base, many continue to teach in the same traditional way in the clinical laboratory: they teach as they have been taught.

Importance

Lindsey et al.[2] state that professional laboratories and students' experience in them will be assuming even more importance in the years ahead. However, they state that an important factor is the quality of experience that students can obtain in the professional laboratory. Yet Sister Zasowska[3] concluded in a study in 1967 that the clinical laboratory experience in nursing tends to be obscurely defined and ambiguously identified. Her study described the overall aspects of the clinical laboratory, but intensive study of what the student *does* in the laboratory has just begun to be made.

The need is to examine the very nature of clinical laboratory activities in nursing education and focus attention on the activities that the teacher provides in nursing programs to make them a real educational opportunity. What, in fact, is a clinical laboratory for? How do teachers of nursing use a clinical laboratory? Because the teacher fashions the learning environment, the focus of this book is on the teacher's point of view. Hopefully, the points raised will give additional insight into the clinical laboratory problems that are often discussed in the nursing literature.

Educators are now beginning to realize the impact of the clinical setting in nursing education. They are concerned about what can be done to make this setting a more effective learning environment. Yet it is questionable whether or not the present methods of teaching in the clinical laboratory are correct or necessary. Is change needed? If so, a change to what?

Before considering change, we should examine the present laboratory activities in light of what they should be to determine whether or not they meet educational criteria. We should examine the laboratory concept and how it applies to nursing education. This approach will answer the complaints of Mildred Montag, Loretta Heidgerken, and other nurse educators that the clinical laboratory activities for nursing students have reflected a "practitioner-" or "worker-" oriented assignment instead of a "learner-" oriented opportunity. This may be a remnant from the apprenticeship training of nurses to the education of nurses in institutions of higher learning.

Hagen[4] asks these questions of nurse educators: "How do you learn about nursing?" "How do you assign students?" "Why do you assign students in the way that you do?" She has not received adequate answers, and she believes that a study is needed in these areas.

Zasowska recommends an appraisal of the effective use of the student's time, of the resources of the educational institution, and of the resources of the community. From the teachers' and the students' standpoint, the most time-consuming aspect of the nursing student's program is the clinical laboratory. A change in the use of this laboratory will result in more efficient and more effective learning.

Schwab,[5] in discussing change, states that empirical study of teaching action is necessary to know what we are doing, what we are not doing, and to what effect, that is, what changes are needed and what changes can be effected in view of costs and the educational effort. This book deals with what teachers of nursing are doing, what they are not doing, and what they might be doing in the clinical laboratory. The kinds of changes suggested flow from both educational theory and widely accepted practices in education for the professions. The original work done on the laboratory concept from which the essential elements were derived is summarized in Appendix A.

Too often in nursing education, changes have been instituted without a sound basis. Clinical laboratory hours have been increased or decreased; student–faculty ratios have been set; and types of clinical laboratory activities have been determined without an investigation of the purpose for the change. According to Lindsey et al.,[6] teachers who take an action research approach are more likely to improve their operations on the basis of evidence than on the basis of opinion or untested hunches. The members of a profession are responsible for making decisions based on study and investigation, not on guesswork or ignorance.

Nurse educators have begun in selected instances to study various approaches to the use of the clinical laboratory in a systematic fashion. Some of these studies are listed in the bibliography at the end of this chapter; others are included in subsequent chapters as they relate to specific considerations under discussion. Such studies have been done from the learner's point of view as well as from that of the faculty members. The perceptions of relevance of clinical activities and the extent of problem-solving exercises have been carefully examined. Whereas the increasing numbers of studies on clinical laboratory in nursing are encouraging, the findings, by and large, point to the need for nurse faculty to be more carefully and consistently guided by sound educational theories and philosophies rather than by past practices to structure clinical activities.

Additionally, nurse educators need to be cognizant of and study the effectiveness and efficiency of selected strategies of clinical teaching. Schwab's recommendations based on costs and the expended educational effort can no longer be ignored by nurse faculty. Costs for and expectations of institutions of higher learning continue to rise. Tuition costs are escalating at an alarming rate, to the point, in fact, of being beyond the reach of many middle-class Americans. And despite increasing revenues to colleges and universities, faculties and administrators are faced with tighter, more austere budgets. At the same time, the consumer is making different and increased demands on higher education. All educators are forced to become more highly accountable to students and society than ever before.

Nurse educators are faced with the same problems and challenges of their faculty colleagues. They are responsible for producing for society a more competent, knowledgeable, skillful practitioner of nursing than has ever been expected in our history, while simultaneously wrestling with the greatest numbers of students and scarcest resources ever. Handling these numbers of students in the clinical laboratory poses the greatest challenge, sometimes even with reductions in faculty positions. For many years, the clinical laboratory environment needed for teaching nursing frequently has been cited as the reason for more faculty, less time, and higher costs to support programs of nursing. These arguments are no longer convincing. So, faculty need to explore strategies for the use of the clinical laboratory in nursing education, with renewed interest and zeal. Ways may be developed that are effective in terms of learning outcomes and cost efficiency. The recommendations made in the following chapters are intended to address both points.

Purpose

The overall function of instruction in the clinical laboratory is to provide students with "real experiences" and the opportunity to discover for themselves modes of practice regardless of whether or not these practices already have been discovered by other practitioners. The clinical laboratory serves as a place for students to learn—learn to transfer knowledge already acquired to practical, dynamic situations. The student is actively raising questions, thinking creatively, and producing purposeful action. The student becomes involved in client activities that require skills of observation, experimentation, and investigation, all aimed toward the solution of health-related problems.

The teacher guides and facilitates student learning activities in the clinical laboratory; the teacher does not teach in the clinical laboratory. The teaching has been done before the use of the clinical laboratory, that is, in the classroom and college laboratory. Relevant activities are orchestrated by the teacher for the student to experience in his or her own fashion. The clinical laboratory is the culminating activity that affords the student the opportunity to practice already acquired intellectual and psychomotor skills—not to acquire the theoretical principles behind the skills. Further, it is the place for students to go beyond what has been learned, to change and adapt approaches to care, and to search for a higher quality of care. Through such use of the clinical laboratory, students discover creative modes of practice and add to present or existing knowledge.

The question among educators is not so much whether or not these points are valued and desired, but how best to achieve them, how to sequence activities, and when to introduce each set of activities. As the various points are explored, an important distinction among widely used terminology needs to be understood. There are a variety of uses of terms in nursing education. To clarify the exact use of these as they relate to nursing education, the following definitions are offered.

LABORATORY. Any place, situation, or set of conditions that is conducive to experimentation, investigation, and observation.

CLINICAL. Based on actual observation and treatment of disease or conditions of life instead of on artificial experimentation or theory.

CLINICAL LABORATORY. An institution, home, or community agency where a nursing student comes in contact with clients for the purpose of acquiring intellectual and psychomotor skills.

COLLEGE LABORATORY. A place on the college campus that is equipped with simulated materials for the nursing student to practice in an artificial instead of a real situation. (No clients are in this setting.)

ACTIVITIES. Specific actions that require active involvement and direct experience by the student—what the student actually *does* in the college laboratory and in the clinical laboratory.

Although the term *patient* is more commonly used among health professionals, the term *client* will be used instead. Patient connotes illness and passivity in relation to determinations about one by health professionals, including the nurse. On the other hand, client connotes just the opposite—a well person as well as an ill person with a very active involvement in decisions affecting his or her health and well-being. Client is deemed a more exacting term in light of the values held by nursing and in terms of the type of people cared for by nurses.

Also, the term *clinical activities* rather than *clinical experiences* is used because the teacher may and should direct activities, but cannot control experiences. The ultimate experiences that result from a set of clinical activities is highly individualized for each student and may remain unknown to the teacher.

Placement in the Curriculum

Schofield and Finnila[7] are not sure whether or not students save time by performing skills for the first time with patients instead of in the college laboratory. Although time is an important aspect in educating nurses, the more basic question is whether or not the clinical laboratory is actually the correct place to teach skills for the first time. The amount of time needed in either setting should be determined as a result of an answer to the basic questions. Where do students learn most effectively? Where do students learn most efficiently?

Unfortunately, too frequently the apprenticeship or worker-oriented programs have been transplanted to the college or university campus. Students are expected to learn through on-the-job training as opposed to actual practice after the acquisition of knowledge and skills in the educational setting. Whereas this latter notion has been accepted by nurse educators, actual practices suggest the contrary. Students are assigned to activities before they have studied the underlying concepts and acquired the relevant skills. The demands and the chance opportunities of the clinical settings take precedence over learning considerations. Even the labels ascribed to our students support the point; they are often called *student nurses* rather than *nursing students*. Very different meanings and expectations are conveyed when the noun is *nurse* rather than *student*.

Nurse faculty are engaged in an academic enterprise and are governed by the same standards as other educators. Therefore, they must accept the responsibility of providing opportunities for students to learn through an educational environment in *every* aspect of their program of study. As Bridgman[8] stated, nursing students should receive the benefits of a genuine college education. To do this, their teachers must explore, understand, accept, and use the essential elements of the laboratory concept. All phases of the program of study, including the clinical laboratory, must be viewed as an educational enterprise. The needs of the learner and the principles of learning and teaching guide the actions of both student and faculty. A progression of learning activities from knowing through application, integration, and synthesis serves as the guide.

Notes

1. Cox, C. Frontiers of nursing in the 21st century: Lessons from the past and present for future directions in nursing education. *International Journal of Nursing Studies*, 1982, *19* (1), 1–9.
2. Lindsey, M. et al. *Inquiry into teaching behavior of supervisors in teacher education laboratories.* New York. Teachers College Press, Teachers College, Columbia University, 1969, p. 253.
3. Zasowska, M. A. *A descriptive survey of factors in the clinical laboratory experience in baccalaureate education for nursing.* Unpublished doctoral dissertation, Teachers College, Columbia University, 1967.
4. Hagen, E. Effective use of clinical experience. Lecture to the Nursing

Education Club. New York: Teachers College, Columbia University, November 15, 1967.

5. Schwab, J. J. The practical: A language for the curriculum. *School Review*, 1969, *78* (1), 15–16.

6. Lindsey, M., et al. *Improving laboratory experiences in teacher education*. New York: Bureau of Publications, Teachers College, Columbia University, 1959, p. 26.

7. Schofield, A. M., & Finnila, M. C. L. A place to explore. *Journal of Nursing Education*, 1967, *6* (3), 3.

8. Bridgman, M. *Collegiate education for nursing*. New York: Russell Sage Foundation, 1953, p. 97.

Bibliography

Adams, E. Frontiers of nursing in the 21st century: Development of models and theories on the concept of nursing. *Journal of Advanced Nursing*, 1983, *8* (1), 41–45.

Allerman, G. A. G., & Britten, M. X. W. *Nursing students' perceptions of the relevance and use of the clinical laboratory in learning the practice of nursing: A twin study*. Unpublished doctoral dissertion, Teachers College, Columbia University, 1974.

Bell, D. E. *Survey of the utilization of curriculum innovations in baccalaureate programs of nursing*. Unpublished doctoral dissertation, St. Louis University, 1979.

Burns, M. E. *Faculty opinions on their academic responsibilities in baccalaureate nursing programs*. Unpublished doctoral dissertation, Teachers College, Columbia University, 1969.

Christy, T. E. *Cornerstone for nursing education*. New York: Teachers College Press, Columbia University, 1969.

Cox, C. Frontiers of nursing in the 21st century: Lessons from the past and present for future directions in nursing education. *International Journal of Nursing Studies*, 1982, *19* (1), 1–9.

Dixon, J. K., & Koerner, B. Faculty and student perceptions of effective teaching in nursing. *Nursing Research*, 1976, *25* (4), 300–305.

Fahy, E. Emerging trends in professional health practice affecting patient care. Paper presented at the Fourth Annual Forum of the New England Council on Higher Education for Nursing. Boston, Massachusets, April 17, 1969.

Glass, H. P. *Teaching behavior in the nursing laboratory in selected baccalaureate nursing programs in Canada*. Unpublished doctoral dissertation, Teachers College, Columbia University, 1971.

Henning, E. *Students' perceptions of clinical laboratory activities in baccalaureate programs in nursing.* Unpublished doctoral dissertation, Teachers College, Columbia University, 1974.

Infante, M. S. *The laboratory concept in baccalaureate education in nursing.* Unpublished doctoral dissertation, Teachers College, Columbia University, 1971.

Infante, M. S. Toward effective and efficient use of the clinical laboratory. *Nurse Educator*, 1981, *6* (1), 16–19.

Lindsey, M. *Improving laboratory experiences in teacher education.* New York: Bureau of Publications. Teachers College, Columbia University, 1959.

Makarem, S. N. H. *Faculty report on the organization and structure of the clinical laboratory experiences of senior students in baccalaureate nursing programs.* Unpublished doctoral dissertaion, Teachers College, Columbia University, 1978.

Mayer, G. G., & Frederickson, K. C. *Problem solving by nursing students: A twin study.* Unpublished doctoral dissertation, Teachers College, Columbia University, 1974.

McCaffery, M. What is the student learning in the clinical laboratory? *Journal of Nursing Education*, 1968, *7* (4), 3–10.

Sanders, F. V. *Nursing faculty's and students' perceptions of the relevance and usage of the clinical laboratory.* Unpublished doctoral dissertation, Teachers College, Columbia University, 1977.

Smith, D. W. Some problems of baccalaureate programs. *American Journal of Nursing*, 1970, *70* (1), 120–123.

Smyth, M. P., & Elder, N. Nursing education curriculums, 1968; Direction or drift? *Nursing Outlook*, 1968, *17* (12), 41–43.

Zasowska, M. A. A. *A descriptive survey of significant factors in the clinical laboratory experience in baccalaureate education for nursing.* Unpublished doctoral dissertation, Teachers College, Columbia University, 1967.

Zungolo, E. *A systems analysis of clinical laboratory experiences in baccalaureate nursing education.* Unpublished doctoral dissertation, Teachers College, Columbia University, 1972.

CHAPTER 2

The Laboratory Concept in a Developing Society

The word *laboratory* is derived from the medieval Latin *laboratorium*, meaning workshop. According to the *Encyclopedia Americana*, the word is used to denote any room or building devoted to experimental investigations in techniques and the sciences. The purpose of the experimentation is to advance man's knowledge of special applications of natural law or of human physiology and mentality. Webster states that, historically, the laboratory was the workroom of the chemist. It was a place devoted to the experimental study of natural science, testing, analyzing, and preparing various chemical materials. The major purpose of the laboratory, then, was clearly for experimentation.

Ancient Concept of the Laboratory

During the first six centuries A.D., the laboratory was primarily a place to make drugs and potions. However, at this time, such practices were frowned on. Consequently, the priests, who were the persons making and using these drugs, carried on secret practices under the guise of their other priestly activities. The place where the drugs were made was simply called a workshop.

Also, there is a long history of using the laboratory for demonstrations and experiments as a combined nonverbal and verbal technique of organized learning. It originated in museum displays or collections of natural curiosities. The first museums of educational material were Greek medical collections that Hippocrates himself was supposed to have used for self-education. Another use of these displays was for mechanical demonstrations and acts of ritual, sorcery, and juggling, either to amuse or to train others to accept some belief.[1] However, it was clear that the laboratory was a place in which to seek new knowledge.

Medieval Patrons of Laboratories

Out of the early laboratories of the first six centuries grew those of the Middle Ages. In this later period, laboratories were devoted to astrology and the making of drugs, potions, and charms. They also became the center of a search for a means to change baser metals into gold. Support was derived from nobles who became patrons of such laboratories, or they were maintained at public expense.

The physical science laboratory was developed in Europe during the time of the American Revolution. The chemical laboratory was developed about 1763.[2] Experimentation and the recording of results were the major activities of these laboratories. The early science experiments were off-shoots of the sixteenth-century metallurgical testing procedures.

In addition to exploration, these laboratories also devoted attention to teaching. This represents a major difference in the use of the laboratory during this period. A search was determined and directed by the scientist; the research was done by the assistants and students. Students thus learned the science and the research process.

During the Middle Ages, various medieval associations, such as those of merchants or various tradesmen, were formed to protect the interests of their members and provide training for the young and newly inducted members. Then the laboratories began to be used to train students in the trades. This development is the beginning of the use of the laboratory in training students for an occupation.

Nineteenth-Century Link Between the Guild and the Professions

Purkinje established a physiological laboratory at Breslau in 1825. His laboratory was among the first to be open to university students. A chemical laboratory was established by Baron von Liebig at the Univeristy of Giessen in the same year. The first physical science laboratories for students were founded about 1846, one at Heidelberg by Philip Gustav Jolly, and one at the University of Glasgow by William Thomson-Lord Kelvin.[3]

During this period, the use of the apprenticeship system of teaching became widely used in the trades and extended into education for the professions. Under this plan, a student (apprentice) attached himself to a master and observed his highly expert work. Gradually, the apprentice attempted to imitate the work of the master under his close supervision.

The apprenticeship system is concisely described by Kohn in an article about the architect, Paolo Soleri. At Cosanti, Arizona, the students apprentice themselves to this dedicated architect. They live and work with him while receiving lodging and some grocery money in return. The students also receive the privilege of executing Soleri's designs. Creativity is encouraged in the apprentices, who are expected to execute the finished drawings in their own style under the direction of the master.

The architect's relationship with his students is close, almost familial, but he refuses to meddle in their personal affairs. "I am not a teacher," he says. "My way is the old way of the *bottega*. The master works and everybody does what the master does. For me that is the only way."[4]

In the apprenticeship system the student remained with the same master for an extended period. The master is recognized by those in his field as being highly expert and greatly accomplished; so the master is a good role model. Finally, although the apprentice is expected to learn through observation of the master's behavior, there is the expectation of ultimately going beyond those accomplishments and becoming a credit to the master.

In the early years of the professions, many prepared their practitioners through an apprenticeship system. At varying stages in their development, each profession eventually moved to a true educational type of preparation in a college or university setting. Qualified teachers used teaching strategies appropriate to a system of higher education. They taught the knowledge and skills basic to their profession. In the laboratory, students practiced the skills of the profession. The college and clinical laboratories gradually were used to teach intellectual skills as well as motor skills.

Modern Use of the Laboratory in Education

In practically all American institutions of higher learning there are laboratories established for the purpose of studying science through experimentation and research. Until modern times, the actual purpose of the laboratory changed very little. At the present time, two major purposes of the laboratory in education for the sciences and the professions can be delineated. First, laboratories are centers for experimentation and research; second, both simulated and real laboratories serve as centers of learning for students. The most significant recent changes have been the introduction of new devices for observation, experimentation, and demonstration. However, these latter developments indicate that the purpose for the laboratory has not changed. Instead, the materials used to carry out the purpose have improved through technology.

At the turn of this century, the Dewey philosophy, "learn by doing," led to the graduate application of the term *laboratory method* in fields other than the pure sciences.[5] This was particularly true in the social sciences. The laboratory method, which stressed the provision of opportunity for the student to apply knowledge to the *real situation* within the system of education, came to be appreciated and used widely. In the past few decades, more specialized training laboratories have been established to train students in the special techniques needed in medicine, engineering, industry, agriculture, and other fields. Computerization of learning laboratories has revolutionized the appearance and the nature of activities that take place there. Yet, the goals of such laboratories remain constant—learning through trial and error. At the present time in education, the laboratory activities consist primarily of involving the student in investigation or experimentation leading toward the solution of a problem. Also, the student participates in activities leading to the acquisition of psychomotor and intellectual skills.

Joyce[6] describes a similar use of the laboratory in modern education. Students pursue an independent type of study whereby they work with materials that are geared to their level of development. Through the use of these materials, the students teach themselves skills and knowledge that are important to them. Independence of learning is believed to lead to independence of practice.

An overall and important function of instruction in the laboratory is to provide students with *real experiences* and to allow them to discover things for themselves, regardless of whether or not these things have already been discovered by others. The laboratory provides students with the opportunity to develop skill in making accurate, orderly observations. In this way, the students discover facts. They also discover how to learn. The importance of allowing students in the laboratory to work through problems themselves to arrive at their own conclusions cannot be overestimated. The advantages will become obvious in their subsequent practice.

When carefully structured and correlated with classroom learnings, laboratory activities result in meaningful experiences for the student. The laboratory provides the vehicle for the student to put knowledge into use. He thus expands his understanding and application of these knowledges. The laboratory also provides the student with the means to acquire motor and intellectual skills systematically.

The Clinical Laboratory in Education
for the Professions

Professions are outgrowths of society's needs or desires for special services. A profession deals with matters that are urgent and significant to people. Education for the professions prepares an individual to provide one or more of these specialized services to society. Combs[7] suggests that the professional who deals with human problems regards himself as an intelligent human being. The professional uses self, knowledge, and the resources at hand to solve the problems under the responsibility of that profession.

Professional education must be directed toward guiding a student in the acquisition of knowledge of self, understanding of the world in which he lives, and knowledge of the particular area of expertise. He must be professionally competent in the practice of skills related to the service rendered. McGlothlin[8] states that a student in a professional program must integrate knowledge and skills into a body of effective procedures that he recalls in order to solve problems assigned to the profession. The clinical laboratory is of tremendous importance in helping the student to integrate learnings and to make the transition from a student to a professional person.

According to Hearn,[9] professional practice is a combination of believing, knowing, and doing. He describes each of these actions.

> To act with professional integrity is to act consistently within a framework of values that is shared generally by the members of a profession. To act with knowledge is to act with an awareness of the rationale and probable consequences of one's action. To act with skill is to exercise such control that one's actions most closely approximates one's intentions."

The beginning skills or the "doings" of a professional practitioner are largely acquired in the clinical laboratory component of the educational program.

McGlothin points out that although the professional curriculum is moving toward greater emphasis on knowledge and less emphasis on the skills of practice, professional programs will continue to have the mastery of some skills as an objective. However, the teaching of skills as ends in themselves, that is, separated from the context in which they will be used, appears to be declining.

Professional education has been described by Fahy[10] as a bridge between the world of thought and the world of action. She believes that the first responsibility of the professional practitioner is competence—competence in skill, but skill that flows from organized knowledge. The clinical laboratory is the place that affords the student in the professions the opportunity to acquire such skill.

The classroom and the college laboratory provide the framework within which learning can take place. The clinical laboratory is the place where the student comes in contact with the client, patient, pupil, or other consumer of his service for the purpose of testing his theories and learning the facts. It is the real world.

In summary, professional education provides the environment of the clinical laboratory in order that the student might master the process of application by being placed in actual situations that require the service of the professional. Under the guidance of a competent faculty member, he is allowed to take the needed action. In addition to applying what he has learned, he may go beyond what he has learned, testing alternatives, recognizing his deficiencies, and gradually gaining new insights into his practice.

With the above in mind, an examination of the clinical laboratory in teacher education, medicine, social work, and nursing was made to determine the common concepts in this part of the educational program of these service-oriented professions. Specific reference is made to highlights of the clinical laboratory that pertain to each of these four professions.

Clinical Laboratory in Teacher Education.   The American Association of Colleges for Teacher Education has defined the clinical laboratory component of the program for teacher education as follows.

> Professional laboratory experiences include all those contacts with children, youth, and adults (through observation, participation and teaching) that make a direct contribution to the understanding of individuals and their guidance in the teacher-learning process.[11]

It has been found that early in the history of teacher education, "direct experience" referred merely to a certain number of hours of practice teaching for persons interested in teacher education. "Professional education" referred to a few practical lessons on schoolkeeping. Through the years, however, the laboratory in teacher education evolved into a meaningful learning situation that provided students with the opportunity to apply theory to practice in a real situation under competent guidance.

Although the definition cited above is acceptable to the teaching profession, Marcella Lawler[12] further defines the word *experience*. "Experience" refers to what happens or occurs internally to the individual. The teacher plans for opportunities for learning instead of for the learning experiences. Although the teacher can plan for the opportunity for experiences, the experience is different for each individual student. The teacher cannot control the student's experience. The teacher cannot provide a predetermined experience. Each student may participate in the same activities, yet have a different experience.

The clinical laboratory in teacher education seems to emphasize the importance of providing a bridge from theory to practice and of having competent guidance for the student teacher while this is being accomplished. The preparation for teaching precedes participation in the clinical laboratory. Courses in general education, content areas of specialization, and methods courses are prerequisites to practice teaching. Tanruther[13] describes the clinical laboratory as the test of all that has gone before. He believes that it gives the prospective teacher the chance to synthesize all that has been learned and to translate it into professional skill.

In discussing the preparation of the person preparing to teach in a college, McGrath[14] says that the college teacher should learn the skills of his craft by performing them under an experienced practitioner. He further states that however extensive and precise the theoretical knowledge, the student really becomes a competent practitioner only after actual use of this knowledge in the practical problems of the classroom. Note that the competent guidance of a master teacher who provides for meaningful activities is imperative. Also imperative is the need for unrestricted observation and experimentation before the student begins to teach and during the actual practicum. The clinical laboratory is a culminating experience. It takes place near the end of the student's educational program.

Clinical Laboratory in Medical Education.   "The word *clinical* derives from the Greek, meaning *of the bed,* and it implies a unique part of clinical teaching in medicine."[15] The words *clinical laboratory* were first used in medical education. In medicine, the learning process involves teacher, student, and patient. It is a form of the case method used by other professions in that it is being directed toward a particular occurrence, set of facts, or situations.

The clinical activities of medical students are designed to help them put their *tools to work.* Knowledge of the chemical, physical, and biological sciences enables the student to gather and evaluate evidence, learn to discriminate between valuable and unessential observations, and weigh subtle implications of organic and functional variations. He learns to reach conclusions that may involve varied and seemingly unrelated factors, and to understand the physical and emotional manifestations associated with ill health.

The medical student collects data by obtaining a history of the patient's illness, examining him, conducting laboratory tests as indicated, and eventually arriving at a diagnosis. This medical diagnosis is discussed with the instructor and other students in order to verify his conclusions. During the early part of the clinical laboratory, the student has no responsibility for treatment. The focus is solely on learning to diagnose. Medical students learn about the course and treatment of all important diseases and their complications and have the opportunity to observe each before they learn to treat them. When a thorough understanding of the health problem has been acquired, the student then learns to take actions to reverse the situation.

The problem-solving approach to the diagnosis and treatment of conditions and the development of judgment in the selection and use of treatment is emphasized. Testing of theories to discover the best modes of treatment is the modus operandi. This approach is practiced through contact with patients in teaching hospitals and clinics and through active participation in small group conferences and discussions.

Observations are expected throughout the program of studies, and the student is given time to make accurate observations. Medical students are not responsible for the care or treatment of patients. Faculty or community physicians carry the responsibility for quality care. Learning is stressed. Caughey[16] states that the student is reminded repeatedly that responsibility for the care of the patients resides in the staff of the university hospital. Close contact with each student is maintained throughout the year by a clinical preceptor. The preceptors meet with their group of students for two hours each week. These students also observe families in the community during a long period and work with a team of other health personnel to provide their care. In each situation, patients know that they are students and not physicians.

Throughout the first phase of clinical instruction, medical students develop only a foundation for their learning through the opportunity to learn certain essentials. To this foundation, the student of medicine must add expertise and competence through specialized and advanced training beyond the formal educational program. While problems in medical education's use of clinical lab exist, aspects of nursing education could benefit from it.

Clinical Laboratory in Education for Social Work.   Educational programs in the field of social work also provide for student activities in real-life situations. The setting for this laboratory may be an office, home, hospital, or community agency. Nevertheless, the student is provided with the opportunity to apply theory to practice in social casework through planned activities with individuals, families, or groups in need of this service.

Hearn[17] describes professional practice as a combination of believing, knowing, and doing. He further itemizes the elements that he believes constitute the learning process in social work or other professions as experiencing, well-ordered empirical inquiry, conceptualizing, testing or verifying theories, concretizing, and communications. The theory that is basic to each of these processes is learned in various courses throughout the program. The verification of the theory is carried out in the clinical laboratory.

The student of social work is encouraged to apply knowledge, understanding, and skill creatively to situations with clients. This is done only when such knowledge and skill has been acquired to the extent that the student is free to depart from the established order of thinking and doing. In such practice the principles remain the same; the activities change. Towle[18] says that such depth of integration occurs through an enduring learning process that is contingent on the conditions of practice set by the professional school. Such an educational system provides a body of principles and concepts for differential use. The process endeavors to set in motion a system of learning that will endure and wax strong throughout the years of professional activity. In short, Towle believes that education for the practice of social work trains for professional self-dependence. Clinical laboratory activities provide for independent action based on theory.

Clinical Laboratory in Nursing Education.   Nursing education has from its inception included the use of the clinical laboratory in its educational programs. During certain stages in its history, and perhaps to a great extent even today, numerous hours have been spent in the clinical laboratory by the student. Like the other professions, nursing believes that the clinical laboratory is an important part of the program, and the profession strives to increase the learning productivity of the student during the hours spent in the laboratory.

Throughout the literature on clinical laboratory in nursing education, the importance of students using the problem-solving method in this setting is stressed. Authors on this subject generally agree that the laboratory is the place to test hypotheses. These hypotheses are arrived at on the basis of knowledge, analysis of past experiences, and educated guesses. The laboratory is a place to learn to apply knowledge. It is a place to be creative. The importance of providing for student participation in the selection of clinical laboratory activities has been widely subscribed to. Yet any number of authors talk about "the selection of patients" for whom the student will care. "Patient selection" instead of the "selection of opportunity for learning" is cited consistently. It is taken for granted that "caring for patients" always constitutes a clinical laboratory assignment in nursing education on each level of the nursing major. "Caring for patients" is believed to be synonymous with learning. The idea that the student is not a nurse but is learning to become a nurse is often forgotten. Herein seems to lie the greatest difference between education for nursing and education for the other professions.

In recent years there have been indications that experimentation has been undertaken by faculty members in nursing programs. These studies explore teacher strategies appropriate to teaching in the clinical laboratory. Some efforts at individualizing instruction and the time spent in the clinical laboratory, as well as using simulated laboratory situations early in the student's program of study, are detailed. Yet the clinical laboratory activities are still centered on patient care instead of on student learning. The faculty member is still portrayed as the supervisor or helper in the situation. To have students so deeply involved in caring for patients at all levels in the program seems to have become the plight of the nurse educator.

Use and Misuse of Clinical Laboratory Activities in Nursing Education

Unlike the other professions, nursing education has had some unique problems in the use of the clinical laboratory for the education of its practitioners. Nursing education has had an historical difficulty in identifying what clinical teaching consists of. Traditionally, the instruction of the hospital school student has been largely service under supervision instead of clinical instruction. There was little or no control by the faculty over instruction. The problems originated in the hospital setting.

For example, during the first part of the twentieth century the nursing student was actually conceived of as a worker instead of as a student. Training was haphazard, poorly organized, and concerned primarily with the development of manual skills and the strict adherence to rules and regulations. The nursing student was taught to obey orders and discouraged from much independent thinking.[19] When baccalaureate programs in nursing were founded, the same teaching strategies were used.

As late as the middle of this century, Bridgman stated that in some baccalaureate schools the clinical experience was still primarily a work instead of a learning situation. Systematic instruction was almost wholly confined to classes. She points out that such an emphasis on service inhibited nursing from using clinical instruction with the same care and effectiveness that medicine and veterinary medicine have achieved.

Even today, such statements are applicable to programs in nursing education. Activities of nursing students in the clinical laboratory center largely on rendering total care to patients. This is true even of laboratory activities early in the program of studies. *Learning* is believed to take place while *caring*. Students carry responsibility for patient care.

Quint[20] questions whether or not the performance expectations of nursing students during their early clinical laboratory experiences are realistic. She points out that medical students have limited contact with patients. Medical students are not responsible for making medical decisions. In contrast, nursing students care for patients from the beginning. They practice the fundamental nursing techniques and carry the rasponsibility for nursing actions relatively quickly. The stress caused young students by this weighty responsibility too soon actually interferes with learning.

Some nurse educators, early in the developmental stages of the profession, understood what the clinical laboratory was all about. Apparently, their ideas were not heeded. Half a century ago, Nutting[21] insisted that nursing students be taught to observe and base their actions on observations. She stressed that the first step for the student was to participate in directed data collection. The need to introduce the student to the processes of nursing care instead of the rendering of care itself was advocated.

Somewhat related to the idea that nursing students learn by caring is the reference in much of the literature to the idea that the system of nursing education during the early part of this century had been an apprenticeship type of preparation. A number of authors on the clinical laboratory in nursing education have referred to the student as an "apprentice" instead of a "learner." Yet some elements of a true apprenticeship are missing. Nursing students have never been attached to a master practitioner. They have inadvertently used a number of practitioners as role models, who may or may not have been master practitioners. Students have been expected to "learn as they go" in a variety of situations. This process more closely approximates the continuing education of an accomplished practitioner of nursing instead of the formal educational process of a learner in a university program or even in an apprenticeship program.

The apprentice "learns by doing." Instead, nursing education had its origins in "doing in order to learn." Trial and error through direct experience and without adequate knowledge of how to test theories was the method used. Zasowska states that nursing education gradually evolved into an apprenticeship. At best, this may be the case. However, it seems to have fallen short of a true apprenticeship, and instead, likens to a worker-type or on-the-job training experience.

In contrast to the image of the dependent, obedient, passive nursing student held in the first part of this century, nurse educators currently strive to produce independent, creative, decisive, assertive thinkers for the practice of nursing. And curiously enough, although beliefs about what the professional ought to be have changed dramatically, the educational strategies used in the clinical laboratory remain amazingly constant, except for the efforts of a few. The educative process of developing a sound thinking person appears to be arbitrary and elusive to many nurse educators. Whereas current objectives of undergraduate nursing programs emphasize creative client care, little or no formal preparation for the process of determining and rendering such care is provided. There is very little evidence of the socialization of nursing students to the norms of behavior associated with the discovery and transmission of new knowledge.

This continuing, atypical use of the clinical laboratory in nursing education, as documented in the literature, and as experienced by faculty and students, has led to the identification of the essential elements of the laboratory concept. Discussion and analysis of these elements suggest a refreshing approach to a redefined use of the clinical laboratory in nursing education.

Notes

1. Smith, K. V., & Smith, M. F. *Cybernetic principles of learning and educational design.* New York: Holt, Rinehart and Winston, Inc., 1966, p. 74.

2. Ibid., p. 76.

3. Laboratory. *Encyclopedia Americana,* 1955, *16,* p. 615.

4. Kohn, S. D. Paolo Soleri thinks very big. *New York Times Magazine,* July 26, 1970, p. 39.

5. Heidgerken, L. E. *Teaching and learning in schools of nursing.* Philadelphia: J. B. Lippincott Company, 1965, p. 431.

6. Joyce, B. *The teacher and his staff: Man, media, and machines.* Washington, D.C.: The National Education Association of the United States, 1967, p. 21.

7. Combs, A. W. *The professional education of teachers.* Boston: Allyn and Bacon, Inc., 1965, p. 8

8. McGlothlin, W. J. *The professional schools.* New York: Center for Applied Research in Education, 1964, p. 2.

9. Hearn, G. *Theory building in social work.* Canada: University of Toronto Press, 1958, p. 1.

10. Fahy, E. *Emerging Trends in Professional Health Practice Affecting Patient Care.* Paper presented at the Fourth Annual Forum of the New England Council on Higher Education for Nursing. Boston, Massachusetts, April 17, 1969.

11. McGeorch, D. M. *Direct experiences in teacher education.* New York: Bureau of Publications, Teachers College, Columbia University, 1953, p. 1.

12. Lawler, M. (Ed.). *Strategies for Planned Curricular Innovation.* New York: Teachers College Press, Columbia University, 1970, p. 17.

13. Tanruther, E. M. *Clinical Experiences in Teaching for the Student Teacher or Intern.* New York: Dodd, Mead and Company, 1967, p. 9.

14. McGrath, E. The preparation of college teachers: Some basic considerations. *Journal of Teacher Education,* 1962, *13* (3), p. 252.

15. McGlothlin, W. J. *Patterns of professional education.* New York: G. P. Putnam's Sons, 1960, p. 86.

16. Caughey, J. L., Jr. Clinical teaching during four years. *Journal of Medical Education*, 1956, *31* (8), p. 530.
17. Hearn, G. *Theory building in social work*. Canada: University of Toronto Press, 1958, p. 1.
18. Towle, C. *The Learner in education for the professions*. Chicago: The University of Chicago Press, 1954, p. 411.
19. Christy, T. E. *Cornerstone for nursing education*. New York: Teachers College Press, Columbia University, 1969, p. 45.
20. Quint, J. C. The hidden hazards in patient assignments. *Nursing Outlook*, 1965, *13* (11), p. 50.
21. Nutting, M. A. *A sound economic basis for schools of nursing*. New York: G. P. Putnam's Sons, 1926, p. 33.

Bibliography

American Association of Teachers Colleges. *School and community laboratory experiences in teacher education*. Oneonta, New York: The Association, 1948.

Association for Student Teaching. *Functions of laboratory schools in teacher education*. Washington, D.C.: The Association, 1955.

Bandman, B., & Guttchen, R. S. *Philosophic essays on teaching*. New York: J. B. Lippincott Company, 1969.

Barrington, T. M. *The introduction of selected educational practices into teachers colleges and their laboratory schools*. New York: Bureau of Publications, Teachers College, Columbia University, for the Institute of Administrative Research, 1953.

Blair, L. C. *An exploration of the nature and function of laboratory experiences in the development of general education courses offered at State Teachers College, Indiana, Pennsylvania*. Unpublished doctoral dissertation, Teachers College, Columbia University, 1953.

Bridgman, M. *Collegiate education for nursing*. New York: Russell Sage Foundation, 1953.

Brown, A. F. *Clinical instruction*. Philadelphia: W. B. Saunders Company, 1949.

Caughey, J. L., Jr. Clinical teaching during four years. *Journal of Medical Education*, 1956, *31*, (8), 530–534.

Combs, A. W. *The professional education of teachers*. Boston: Allyn and Bacon, Inc., 1965.

Conference on the role of the laboratory school in teacher education. Proceedings of Conference held at P. K. Yong Laboratory School, College of Education, University of Florida, Gainesville, Florida, November 23–25, 1958.

Cottrell, D. P., (Ed.). *Teacher education for a free people*. Oneonta, New York: The American Association of Colleges for Teacher Education, 1956.

Cummer, C. L. *Manual of clinical laboratory methods.* Philadelphia: Lea & Febiger, 1922.

Dewey, J. *Democracy and education.* New York: The Macmillan Company, 1916.

———. *Experience and education.* New York: The Macmillan Company, 1938.

———. *How we think.* Boston: D. C. Heath and Company, 1933.

———. The relation of theory to practice in education. *Association for Student Teaching Bulletin,* 1962, No. 17.

Dworkin, M. S. *Dewey on education.* New York: Teachers College Press, Columbia University, 1959.

Flanders, N. A. Integrating theory and practice in teacher education. *Forty-Fourth Yearbook of the Association for Student Teaching,* Dubuque, Iowa: William C. Brown Company, 1965.

Forbes, W. C. *The laboratory experience in science for general education.* Unpublished doctoral dissertation, Teachers College, Columbia University, 1949.

Fritz, E. L. *Faculty selection, appointment, and promotion in collegiate nursing programs.* Unpublished doctoral dissertation, Teachers College, Columbia University, 1965.

Goldhammer, R. *Clinical supervision: Special methods for the supervision of teachers.* New York: Holt, Rinehart & Winston, 1969.

Goodlad, J. I. An analysis of professional laboratory experiences in the education of teachers. *New developments, research, and experimentation in professional laboratory experience.* Edited by the Association for Student Teaching, Cedar Falls, Iowa: Association for Student Teaching, 1964, 32–42.

Hearn, G. *Theory building in social work.* Canada: University of Toronto Press, 1958.

Jaderborg, E. H. *Professional laboratory experiences on the secondary school level in the teacher education program of Bethany College (Kansas).* Unpublished doctoral dissertation. Teachers College, Columbia University, 1966.

Jensen, D. M. *Clinical instruction and its integration in the curriculum.* St. Louis: C. V. Mosby Company, 1952.

Lambertson, E. C. *Education for nursing leadership.* Philadelphia: J. B. Lippincott Company, 1958.

McGeoch, D. M. *Direct experiences in teacher education.* New York: Bureau of Publications, Teachers College, Columbia University, 1953.

McGlothlin, W. J. *Patterns of professional education.* New York: G. P. Putnam's Sons, 1960.

———. *The professional schools.* New York: Center for Applied Research in Education, 1964.

McGrath, E. C. The ideal education for the professional man. *Education for the professions.* Sixty-first Yearbook of the National Society for the Study of Education, Part II. Edited by N. L. Henry, Chicago: University of Chicago Press, 1962.

————. The preparation of college teachers: Some basic considerations. *Journal of Teacher Education*, 1962, *13* (3), 247–252.

Means, J. H. The clinical training of the medical student. *Education for professional responsibility*. Pittsburgh: The Carnegie Press, 1948, p. 116.

Nutting, M. A. *A sound economic basis for schools of nursing*. New York: G. P. Putnam's Sons, 1926.

Oskamp, S. *The relationship of clinical experience and training methods to several criteria of clinical prediction*. Washington: American Psychological Association, 1962.

Pellegrino, E. D. Human values and the medical curriculum. *Journal of the American Medical Association*, 1969, *209* (9), 1349–1353.

Perrodin, A. F. *Teachers who guide professional laboratory experiences: Status, functions, and factors of satisfaction and dissatisfaction*. Unpublished doctoral dissertation, Teachers College, Columbia University, 1952.

Pfefferkown, B. *Clinical education in nursing*, New York: The Macmillan Company, 1932.

Phenix, P. H. *Realms of meaning*. New York: McGraw-Hill Book Company, 1964.

Rivlin, H. N. Theory underlying professional laboratory experience. *Theoretical bases for professional laboratory experiences in teacher education*. Forty-fourth Yearbook of the Association for Student Teaching, Dubuque, Iowa: William C. Brown Company, Inc., 1965.

Rogers, M. *Educational revolution in nursing*. New York: The Macmillan Company, 1961.

Ronneberg, C. E. *Laboratory approach to the physical sciences: A project manual*. Boston: Houghton Mifflin Company, 1965.

Schwab, J. J. *Biology teachers' handbook*. New York: John Wiley and Sons, Inc., 1963.

————. The practical: A language for curriculum. *School Review*, 1969, *78*, (1), 1–23.

Smith, B. O., & Ennis, R. H. (Eds.). *Language and concepts in education*. Chicago: Rand McNally and Company, 1961.

Smith, K. V., & Smith, M. F. *Cybernetic principles of learning and educational design*. New York: Holt, Rinehart & Winston, Inc., 1966.

Stratemeyer, F. B., Forkner, H. L., McKim, M. G., & Passow, A. H. *Developing a curriculum for modern living*. New York: Bureau of Publications, Teachers College, Columbia University, 1957.

Stratemeyer, F. B., Forkner, H. L., McKim, M. G., Passow, A. H., & Lindsey, M. *Working with student teachers*. New York: Teachers College Press, Columbia University, 1958.

Taba, H. *Curriculum development: Theory and practice*. New York: Harcourt, Brace and World, Inc., 1962.

Tanruther, E. M. *Clinical experiences in teaching for the student teacher or intern*. New York: Dodd Mead and Company, 1967.

Towle, C. *The learner in education for the professions.* Chicago: The University of Chicago Press, 1954.

Turner, E. L., Wiggins, W. S., Shepherd, G. R., Sringall, A. N., & Tipner, A. Medical education in the United States and Canada. *Journal of the American Medical Association,* 1956, *161* (17), 1637–1678.

Vocalis, J., & Sheriff, M. *Laboratory experiences prior to student teaching in the pre-service program in childhood education at Teachers College, Columbia University.* Unpublished doctoral dissertation, Teachers College, Columbia University, 1961.

CHAPTER 3

Essential Elements of the Laboratory Concept and Their Application in Nursing Education

The essential elements of the laboratory concept are identified and discussed in terms of the very nature of a clinical laboratory and its proper use in nursing education. These elements emerged as a result of an investigative study of laboratory teaching, its methods, and techniques. A summary of this study is found in the Appendix. The writings on the use of the laboratory in educational programs, and especially the clinical laboratory in the professions, embody this laboratory concept. The ultimate purpose of an in-depth view of the essential elements of this concept is to determine the type of activities in which the learner should be involved in the clinical laboratory in nursing education.

Each of the elements is developed in terms of its major components. That is, the essential types of student or faculty activities that comprise each element are discussed and illustrated. These components resulted from answers derived from the following questions.

1. What is the purpose of a clinical laboratory?
2. What does a teacher guide a student to do in the laboratory?
3. What type of environment should be provided for the student in the clinical laboratory?

4. What common concept(s) is/are used by nursing, teaching, medicine, and social work?

The essential elements of the clinical laboratory that emerged are as follows.

1. Opportunity for client contact.
2. Objectives for activities.
3. Competent guidance.
4. Individuation of activities.
5. Practice for skill learning, both motor and intellectual.
6. Encouragement of critical thinking.
7. Opportunity for problem solving.
8. Opportunity for observation.
9. Opportunity for experimentation.
10. Development of professional judgment or decision making.
11. Encouragement of creative abilities.
12. Provision for transfer of knowledge.
13. Participation in integrative activities.
14. Use of the team concept.

These essential elements should be embodied in the design of clinical laboratory activities in nursing just as they are evident in those of other professions. The overall goal, of course, is to develop a mode of thinking and behaving in the nursing student that will manifest itself consistently in the actions of the practicing professional after graduation, that is, make sound professional judgments, test creative approaches to care, make astute observations.

To accomplish this goal in nursing education, the faculty member and the student need to engage in planned activities appropriate both to a teacher and a learner. Each party in the teaching–learning process carries distinct responsibilities. To more clearly delineate the responsibilities of each, the essential elements have been classified into three categories: teacher responsibility centered; learner centered; and other centered. The categorization emerges as follows.

Category	*Essential Element*
Teacher centered	Type of client contact
	Objectives
	Competent guidance
	Individuation

Category	Essential Element
Learner centered	Skill learning
	Critical thinking
	Problem solving
	Observation
	Experimentation
	Professional judgment
	Creativity
	Transfer of knowledge
	Integrative activities
Other centered	Team concept

The *other centered* category refers to the interaction with other health team members that is so essential to learning the practice of nursing. A role for both the teacher and the learner is inherent in this category.

Much of the discussion of each of the essential elements in the remainder of this chapter addresses the component parts of the elements. Directly or indirectly, the development of each element deals with variations of the use of the element in clinical laboratories in nursing education. Three possible variations serve as the structure for the discussion: positive (the desired educational approach), mixture (a middle-of-the-road blend of the educational and on-the-job training approach with much left to chance), and negative (on-the-job training approach). Table 3.1 depicts the typical type of activity characteristic of that particular element, category, and point on the range of variations. It should serve as a valuable point of reference as each element is subsequently explored.

Opportunity for Client Contact

Client contact is the heart of the student's activities in the clinical laboratory in nursing education. Clinical laboratory activities provide an opportunity for learning in the kinds of situations in which the learners will continue to perform as practitioners.[1] A strength in nursing education has been that nurse educators realize the importance of student contact with the real situation in order that they may be adequately prepared for future roles. All learnings in nursing programs are included for the ultimate application to nursing care needs of clients. Other professions such as business and engineering are becoming more cognizant of the value of the student contact with their clientele during their educational program. Nursing cannot and will not lose sight of this valuable set of learnings, but is striving to improve its effectiveness.

Client contact is necessary but, on the other hand, the clinical laboratory

TABLE 3.1. Essential Elements Organized into Categories and Postulated Range of Variations[a]

Categories of Emphasis	Essential Elements	Postulated Range of Variations		
		Positive	Mixture	Negative
Teacher responsibility-centered	Type of client contact	Apply knowledge to care	Care and knowledge	How to care
	Objectives	Clearly stated educational objective	Vague objective	Lack of educational objective
	Competent guidance	Teach to (active learning; fosters independence)	Teach how (some active—some passive)	Tell to (passive learning; fosters dependence)
	Individuation	Student-initiated activities	Teacher-directed activities	Agency-directed activities
Learner centered	Skill learning	Professional training aimed at competence	Technical training aimed at skill formation with limited knowledge	Habit formation aimed at rapid repetition
	Critical thinking	Promotes	Stifles	Inhibits
	Problem solving	Activities contain some level of uncertainty	Activities involve repetitive tasks	Cut-and-dried routine tasks
	Observation	Observes to learn	Observes while giving care	Lack of observation
	Experimentation	Tests theories	Plans and gives client care	Follows routine
	Professional judgment	Decision-making process used	Needs direction to act	Follows orders strictly
	Creativity	Freedom to exploration and expression	Limited freedom	Follows standard procedures
	Transfer of knowledge	Translates theory into practice	Applies few principles	No transfer—follows directions
	Integrative activities	Maximum knowledge and/or skill	Minimal knowledge and/or skill	Lack of knowledge and/or skill
Other centered	Team concept	Team activities practiced	Team activities by chance rather than by design	Lack of team activities

[a]Modification of Kluckhohn-Strodtbeck Model for Classifying of Basic Value Orientations from Florence Kluckhohn and Fred Strodtbeck, *Variations in Value Orientations* (New York: Row, Peterson and Company, 1961), p. 437.

should be used only when it furnishes the best means of goal achievement. It should be used only when that goal cannot be accomplished in the classroom or college laboratory. In nursing education, the clinical laboratory should always involve contact with clients. It should be used. *only* when client interaction is necessary for the student to accomplish a learning objective. Perhaps the crucial consideration is that the type of client contact desired for students determines the nature of the situation in which activities occur.

Rogers[2] writes that laboratory courses in nursing must reflect preceding theoretical content and be consistent with the philosophy and objectives of higher education. They also must provide an opportunity for the use of intellectual operations in meeting health needs. The emphasis in the clinical laboratory should not be on *how to care*, but on *how to apply knowledges to care* for clients. Caring is not synonymous with learning. Actual client situations are used to provide students the opportunity to practice in the real situation. Selected aspects of care serve as the basis for the practice. The theory underlying the practice must be understood and the readiness for the application of the theory to the practice must be assessed by the teacher.

It would follow then that the purpose of teachers of nursing who use the clinical laboratory for student activities should be precisely stated. The accomplishment of a skill objective for a course does not automatically lead to the clinical laboratory activity of students giving care to clients. The skill can be practiced without the attendant care being administered by the student. Moreover, students need not be assigned to practice a skill or give complete care to clients for a prescribed number of hours in order to learn how to care. Freedom and flexibility of the time afforded each student in the college and clinical laboratory should enhance learning. Some students require more time than others to acquire a skill; both types of students should be afforded the chance to determine how long it requires them to learn a set of activities. Assigning all students a four-hour laboratory on a given day at a given time does not necessarily contribute to optimal learning for all students, particularly if much of that time is spent giving routine care to clients.

The skills required to give segments of that care should be acquired first in the college laboratory. Clinical laboratory activities would follow at a later date. In some instances, client contact can be most valuable to beginning students, especially for data collection on a specific problem. However, four hours spent giving routine care to clients to collect specific data that would be acquired in a 15-minute interview is a misuse of academic time and credit. Hence, the difference in laboratory assignments is striking. Student learning instead of client care always must be kept as the focus of clinical laboratory activities by nurse educators. The selection of clients and laboratory time and length should be made on the basis of the learners' needs rather than on the clients' needs.

For example, learning about care of the person on a lowered level of consciousness has many facets. Learning the manifestations of an increase in intracranial pressure, noting the similarities and differences among these manifestations between the person who has an intracranial tumor and the person who has an intracranial hemorrhage, knowledge of the type of skin care needed under such circumstances, and knowledge of the means of keeping a patent airway are all acquired in the classroom and in the college laboratory before client contact. Time and attention is needed to learn the manifestations of the cause of the problem, to deal with the client behaviors, and to insure comfort and safety. Client contact affords opportunity to practice each component of care without the demands of rendering total care to the client.

But later, the culmination of this learning is in the client setting when the student needs to see and cope with these real-life situations and learns to apply knowledge to practice in order to render care. The differentiation of the above activities is learned through classroom discussions, viewing media on the subject, reviewing appropriate readings, and practicing nursing interventions in a simulated setting. The clinical setting is utilized only when the mentioned activities are assimilated to the point where the student can make inferences and apply them to a real situation.

Objectives for Activities

An objective should be stated clearly to the student for each laboratory session. Bruner[3] states that there is a very crucial matter about acquiring any skill. The goal must be plain; students must have a sense of where one is going in any given instance of activity. He goes on to say that in the formal education setting there is a need for more emphasis on making clear the purpose of every exercise, every lesson plan, every unit, every term, and every education. It is essential that the learner understands the reason for and goal of each clinical laboratory. Thus, each session must be carefully structured in terms of its objective, and it must be an integral part of the course. To teach a skill without explaining its context in the total structure is an uneconomical use of time.

Most students have difficulty translating a set of course objectives to the context of the clinical activities on their own accord. Specific laboratory objectives that flow from the course objectives need to be specified by the teacher. Courses should be arranged so that there are logical, sequential sets of activities from one course to the next.

The learner also needs to receive feedback on each objective. In addition to knowing the goal one is trying to reach, the exercise of skill is governed by an intention and feedback mechanism whereby the learner knows what he has achieved thus far. Knowledge of results tends to encourage further attempts to achieve. Some feedback should be teacher provided; some should be self-determined by the learner.

The clinical laboratory should be only one of a variety of available settings used to accomplish objectives. The clinical laboratory should be selected only when the objective cannot be met in the classroom or college laboratory. Otherwise, much valuable time of the teacher, student, and even the client can be wasted. When carefully planned, each hour in clinical laboratory becomes more meaningful and is directed toward a specific goal achievement. Achievement of objectives becomes obvious and enjoyable; students become highly motivated to tackle the next set of objectives. The laboratory experience is a composite activity that in and of itself has no justification in the educational program. Its value depends on the extent to which it facilitates learning of concepts and principles transferable to other situations.[4]

It cannot be assumed that students learn significant facts and techniques by mere exposure to the clinical laboratory. Hanson[5] writes that "learning by experience" is employed to mean that by having any experience, we *always* learn by that experience. He believes that the idea that any experience will produce learning is often the reverse face of the modern educational coin. So it is maintained that selectivity and specificity of the environment used for the accomplishment of objectives by the learner is essential in educational programs.

The selectivity of activities can be directed by the specific objectives set forth. The specificity of the environment is another point that deserves the attention of nurse educators. It does not necessarily follow that the hospital is the best setting for the achievement of laboratory activities. The hospital affords an opportunity to practice a myriad of activities involved in rendering acute care in crisis situations. So the general hospital is an invaluable setting and an oft used one. However, a number of psychomotor skill objectives can better be met in precrisis or postcrisis settings in which most people spend most of their lives. Such settings for practice include the following:

Category	Essential Element
Institutions	General hospitals
	Nursing homes
	Rehabilitation centers
	Hospices
	Psychiatric hospitals
Community settings	Homes
	Schools
	Mental health centers
	Health professional offices
	Business and industrial centers
	Day care centers
	Senior citizen centers
	Leisure settings—camps, resorts, cruise ships

Professional students of nursing need to be free to have exposure to a wide variety of settings, and even to move among settings when appropriate to accomplish an objective.

Some examples of course objectives, clinical laboratory objectives, and suggested settings for practice are presented in Table 3.2. Each of the three course objectives are isolated entities and are not intended to serve as a sequence of course objectives.

In each of the situations in Table 3.2 the actual language of the objective should correspond to the concepts of the conceptual framework used by the school or department. Students and faculty should decide on what activities

TABLE 3.2. Course Objectives, Laboratory Objectives, and Settings

Course Objectives	Laboratory Objective(s)	Settings
Measures vital signs of selected clients	Measures body temperature of clients in three accepted ways	General hospital Nursing home Home School Clinic
	Determines heart rate of clients through three accepted means	
	Measures blood pressure using two accepted means	
	Compares and contrasts findings in measurements	
	Records findings accurately	
Maintains skin integrity	Identifies potential pressure points	Nursing home General hospital Rehabilitation centers Home
	Changes position regularly	
	Positions body in proper alignment	
	Administers preventive skin care	
	Administers therapeutic skin care as indicated	
	Compares and contrasts findings according to age of client, condition, and resources	
	Records findings completely and accurately	
Cares for person with electrolyte imbalance	Observes skin turgor of persons with electrolyte imbalance	General hospital Nursing home
	Interprets blood studies in light of normal values	
	Relates vital signs to improvement or regression of condition	
	Plans dietary intake according to general condition and needs	
	Administers and regulates intravenous solutions accurately	

are practiced in the college laboratory and to what extent. When a certain degree of skill and confidence has been acquired, the student proceeds to practice selected objectives in the clinical laboratory.

What does all of this mean to nursing education? It is not enough for teachers merely to state broad skill objectives for a course. More specific objectives for each laboratory session must be clear to the nursing student. Teacher and student must know exactly what is to be accomplished through specific activities within a given laboratory period. Suggested settings for practice should be discussed. Also, the time spent by the student in the laboratory should be for the accomplishment of that objective and only for that objective. Too often in nursing education, the objectives are too complex. Expectations are stated in terms of a semester instead of a week or a month. The student is unclear as to the goals of each laboratory and tends to lose sight of the trees for the forest.

In addition to clearly stating a laboratory objective, the teacher *must* communicate to the students when each objective is to be accomplished. The time should be specific, but not inflexible. For example, objective number 1 should be achieved within two to four weeks.

To provide the much needed feedback for students, nurse faculty should schedule conferences regularly. Through individual and group conferences, the learner, with the guidance of the teacher, should examine how the objectives have or have not been accomplished. The conference should concentrate on what was accomplished and what was learned, not on whether the student enjoyed the experience or not. At the same time, goals should be set for future activities in relation to the next set of objectives.

It is essential that teachers of nursing attempt to use the clinical laboratory more selectively. It is important to scrutinize skill objectives to determine if the learner can accomplish them in a setting other than the clinical laboratory. If an objective can be met in the classroom, at a seminar, or through individual or group practice in a college laboratory, then it is totally unnecessary to use time in the clinical laboratory to learn that task. This would be unfair to the student's learning and to the patient's right to privacy and expert care.

Competent Guidance

The role of the teacher in learning is crucial. From time to time teachers need to reexamine their strategies and motives. Stratemeyer[6] has written that what is really learned and what goals are actually realized are determined as much by the way in which a selected experience is guided as by its nature. To properly guide the learning of a student, the teachers should be specialists both in the subject matter that they are teaching and in the field of education. This concept is equally true in the laboratory as in the classroom. "The clinical laboratory in the professions is a center of inquiry, and a range of specialists should be available to guide this inquiry."[7] The quality of experience that students have in the laboratory is determined largely by the expertise of those who provide the guidance. Expertise applies to subject matter and an understanding of how to use a clinical laboratory. The expertise can be provided by the faculty members and the practitioners in the setting as resource persons or as preceptors.

To begin with, the central activity of these teachers must be seen as teaching. In the past, the practice of placing undue weight on the overseeing, managing, directing, and assessing functions has, according to Lindsey,[6] resulted in too little emphasis being placed on the actual functions of teaching, that is, guiding, supporting, stimulating, and facilitating. In the laboratory, students must be urged to learn about a subject and to gain a concept of themselves as future practitioners. The teacher facilitates that learning by designing appropriate activities in appropriate settings and allowing the student to experience it. This does not mean that the teacher oversees and manipulates the experience.

The student also can benefit from the demonstrated expertise of expert practitioners in the setting. Their ongoing development of psychomotor skills and professional attitudes, with a cognitive base for both, can serve as the model practice to which the student aspires. Practitioners should serve as resource persons to students and faculty; some practitioners could serve as preceptors to undergraduate and graduate students. Chapter 7 deals with the topic of preceptors in greater detail.

A permissive attitude is necessary in the clinical laboratory. The atmosphere should be one of a nonpunitive, nonjudgmental nature. Value judgments are made as to right and wrong, but the teacher should plan to allow for errors on the part of the learner and then direct the learners to become their own self-correctors. Instead of judging the student's practice, the teacher should assist the student in investigating his own practice and leave the valuing process and the decision to change to the student. During this process, the teacher is available to assist the student in making changes and to set the level of thinking practiced by the students. This latter activity, however, does not and probably should not take place in the clinical setting but rather in individual conferences on the campus. McClelland[8] proposes that the more an individual keeps a record of his own progress toward achieving goals to which he is committed, the more the newly formed motive is likely to influence future thoughts and actions. Perhaps such a record could be used by both teacher and student to examine findings and set new directions.

The overall objective of the teacher is to direct the learner to become self-sufficient. The teacher makes the learning process safer for the student through guidance, rather than through direction. The teacher shows the student the way to approach problem solving based on knowledge in such a way that practice can proceed independently. Otherwise, "the result of instruction is to create a form of mastery that is contingent upon the perpetual presence of a teacher."[9] This infers that the teacher should not impose his will on the student. Instead, in the clinical laboratory, students are provided with the opportunity to broaden the use of their own knowledge in a specialized field with freedom and without restriction. The student becomes actively engaged in learning and is not the passive recipient of knowledge from the teacher.

Laboratory procedures sometimes can be too detailed by teachers. If so, they deprive the student of intellectual challenge. The teacher should not explain every step in a procedure. The teacher should not stand at the student's elbow prompting every step. Teaching students to practice instead of telling them how to practice develops stable patterns of action as opposed to orders aimed at securing immediate compliance. Gagné[10] says that guidance may vary in amount or completeness, but it should always fall short of describing the solution itself. Guidance should inform the learner of the goal of his activity and the basic principles inherent in achieving that goal. It should not limit the range of hypotheses that might be entertained in achieving a solution.

The teacher in the clinical laboratory in nursing should provide real situations to which students can apply acquired knowledges; provide the opportunity for students to present reasoned arguments to her as well as others; support them with knowledge that she possesses; and show confidence in the students' ability to master the situations they face. Guidance should be directed at leading the student to a freedom without restrictions.

Some teachers make the error of providing too much concern and too much information for the sake of being practical and providing for an immediate need of a patient. However, it should be remembered that unless the process has been intellectualized by the student, the retention of such knowledge becomes temporary, and the likelihood of its future use becomes negligible. Moreover, the process by which to arrive at a judgment was not reinforced through use.

Traditionally, nurse faculty members have been overly concerned for the activities of students in the clinical laboratory. This has often occurred under the excuse of providing for the safety of the patient. Teachers fear that students will make an error that will jeopardize the life of a patient. Low faculty–student ratios have been jealously guarded and have resulted in exorbitantly expensive education. However, if these teachers were to accept the fact that true guidance assumes competence in knowledge about the skill or skills to be performed, such fears would be alleviated. Negatively speaking, students should not be in situations in which they lack the knowledge needed to practice and consequently can make fatal errors. In fact, in the method being proposed, the student is expected to be quite knowledgeable and skillful in the clinical laboratory activities assigned, so the probability of error should be less likely. Independence of practice on the part of the student is more reasonable. Guidance assumes a thorough knowledge of the problem solving process. Hence, the concept of guidance assumes that specific directions for giving care and its expected outcomes will *not* be given by the teacher. Low student–faculty ratios would become less necessary.

Perhaps the initial feelings of inadequacy of baccalaureate and associate degree graduates and their fears of being unable to practice skillfully and independently are related to the very close supervision by faculty members that they had during their clinical laboratory activities. To continue to provide these students with little opportunity to develop self-confidence simply perpetuates this problem.

Teachers of nursing should use appropriate evaluation tools to determine that knowledge basic to skills has been learned. Adequate provision should be made for independent learning and practice in the multimedia laboratory and the simulated clinical laboratory. But then students must be allowed the freedom to observe, plan, test, and evaluate their activities in the clinical laboratory without the teacher hovering over them. This would enable teachers of nursing in the clinical laboratory to experience less frantic and fatiguing days. Their time and energy could actually be used for teaching and the time and energy of students could be used for learning. In the field of teaching and learning, leisurely use of time is not a luxury but a necessity. The only provision is that all activities should be goal directed.

Teachers of nursing must guard against a student's inquisitiveness about the manifestations of a health problem being overridden by the need to attend to the hygienic needs of a person who "has to be ready for x-rays at nine a.m." How often have teachers said to students, "We can discuss that after you complete the bath"? Both teachers and students must focus on learning at all times.

This discussion of competent guidance does not infer that the faculty member is never in the clinical laboratory with students. Quite the contrary. But it does force the teacher to examine *teaching activities* in those settings, as well as permit the student a high degree of independence while there. Also, the teacher becomes more selective about when and where and why his or her presence is warranted.

Individuation of Actitivies

Clinical laboratory experiences should be individualized, because they are personal, ego-involving experiences. The experiences vary in value and quality according to individual needs, interests, and abilities. Consequently, the needs, values, and goals of each student should be taken into consideration by the teacher in planning for the nature of and time for laboratory activities. Blair[11] describes this phenomenon succinctly when she states, "A laboratory experience is a personal experience; nothing can be substituted for it. No one but the person who recognizes the problem and is vitally concerned about its solution can realize maximum learning from a direct experience." The values to be derived from a singular experience will vary from student to student.

The problems that the individual learner meets in the laboratory should be immediate and important to him, so that the desire to find the solution to problems presented to him will motivate him to study and inquire into the factors involved. Although the activities might vary according to individual needs, the objectives or goals remain the same. In support of the need for the individuation of all learning activities, Dewey[12] states that the sound educational experience involves, above all, continuity and interaction between the learner and what is learned. On the other hand, he cautions that teachers should avoid the other extreme, which involves inchoate curriculum, excessive individualism, and a spontaneity that is a deceptive index of freedom. It is the responsibility of the teacher, then, to provide structure for the clinical laboratory activities, while guiding each student in the selection and attainment of his goals. In this way the outcomes will be desirable and measurable. For, as Pellegrino[13] writes, "the real test is not the ability of all students to pass the same kind of examination, but rather that each student be evaluated in the pathway he has selected, that is, the one he professes and intends to proclaim in society."

Whereas clinical laboratory activities are personally undertaken, the student should participate in the selection of the learning activities. In fact, clinical laboratory activities often should be personally initiated. In his writing on the acquisition of skills, Bruner holds that teachers would benefit from sharing the process of education with the learner, because there are few things as exciting as sensing in which direction one is trying to go, what one is trying to obtain, and then making progress toward these goals. The excitement of a learner who has attained objectives through his own stated activities brings much satisfaction to a teacher. Because the goals and needs of each student are individual and the experience that is gained is different for each individual, it would be fallacious to suppose that the exposure of all students to the same or even similar activities will result in similar learning.

Learning in the clinical laboratory does not occur as a result of exposure, instead, the provision of activity for the student is to be carefully planned along his identified needs.

Furthermore, not all activities that are desired to achieve a specific objective can be afforded all students. For a variety of reasons, the need for some psychomotor skills, such as urinary catheterization, has been reduced. Rather than fret about the scarcity of such activities, therefore, the use of media and simulated situations and the sharing of students in clinical conferences are enhanced. Other techniques using the same principles, such as asepsis, are arranged for. Individuation of student activities obviates the "sameness" so often aspired to for nursing students and a seeming liability can actually be turned into an asset.

Finally, the individuation of clinical laboratory activities applies to the time spent at each laboratory session. The duration of each period in the clinical laboratory should be long enough to enable the learner to gain adequate skills and understanding, but not so long as to waste time or be repetitious. The time needed in the clinical laboratory will vary for each student because each student learns at a different rate. Setting specific hours for clinical laboratory activities for all students refutes the concept of individuation.

Providing for such individuation is a tremendous undertaking for teachers, especially when large numbers of students are involved. However, it is well worth the effort. Dictating hours or setting is not acceptable or productive, regardless of the reason. Zasowska has written that circumscribing an experience by clock hours and limiting it to a location favored by geographic proximity to the campus may be an administrative necessity, but it is by no means the sole basis for the determination of external limits.

Problems associated with providing for individuation in laboratory experiences are numerous. They involve time to know the learner; time to locate suitable activities; and to arrange and follow through on the learnings. "Whatever the problems, arising from whatever sources, and whatever their magnitude, ways must be found to provide more adequate opportunity than is now available for each individual to progress at his own rate and style."[14]

For example, selected days and times may be designated in a semester schedule for laboratory practice. This time should be free of other course and conference commitments. So typically, most students will use say, Tuesdays and Thursdays for laboratory. And minimal laboratory hours should be set in each course, for example, each student is to spend a minimum of 12 hours per week in the laboratory settings. However, the most able students may spend 12 hours while the slower learner spends 16 hours to achieve the same objectives. One student may choose morning hours to have the best chance of conferring with other health team members, while another student may choose evening hours to confer with family members. Weekends may be preferable to mature students and students with advanced standing due to personal as well as professional responsibilities. The choice of hours should be suggested by students in consultation with the faculty member. Joint decisions should be made.

When applied to nursing education, the concept of individuation of activities in the clinical laboratory implies that each student may approach a particular type of patient problem in a different manner. The problems must be meaningful and the choices differ from student to student. This entire concept is based on the belief that each person has unique abilities and, therefore, has unique contributions to make. Also, each person learns in a different way and at a different pace.

On the other hand, a laissez faire attitude is *not* being advocated. Objectives to be accomplished by clinical laboratory activities are determined by the nurse faculty member. The teacher alone knows what the student should learn. Specific clinical laboratory activities should be personally initiated by the student. How a student learns should be planned jointly by the student and teacher. A wide variety of activities may usually be enumerated to accomplish a goal or objective. To suggest that all students must perform the same activities in a given amount of time is narrow in perspective. In summary, the same objectives need to be accomplished by all students, but differing activities to accomplish these objectives are to be encouraged.

For example, one student of nursing may be interested in spending more time on identifying the problems of and care needed by the elderly; another on the health needs of children. But each may be learning the process of assessment in nursing. Faculty members should permit time and actually arrange for students to inquire into these areas. Also, the faculty members should guide the students to clinical laboratory settings and activities that would satisfy their interest and increase their knowledge and skills in these particular areas.

Practice for Skill Learning

The acquisition of skills continues to be an important objective in professional programs. In these programs there is focus on teaching both the motor and intellectual skills needed to render a specialized service to society. One cannot be emphasized to the exclusion of the other. The clinical laboratory provides the setting in which the learner can practice these skills with the aim of achieving competence in performance for the undergraduate; the graduate student strives for the level of proficiency and mastery.

In all instances, the practice of motor and intellectual skills should be preceded by prerequisite knowledges and understanding. This idea is well documented in the literature. Ryle[15] writes:

. . . the operation which is characterized as intelligent must be preceded by
an intellectual acknowledgment of these rules or criteria; that is, the agent
must first go through the internal process of avowing to himself certain
propositions about what is to be done ("maxims," "imperatives" or "reg-
ulative propositions" as they are sometimes called); only then can he execute his performance in accordance with these dictates. He must preach to
himself before he can practice.

The need for prerequisite knowledge is true not solely for the practice of
intellectual skills, but also for the practice of motor skills. Laboratory procedures not only train the individual to use his eyes and ears in observation,
but also provide practice in motor skills. Motor or physical activities also
require intellectual activities if the aim is the acquisition of skill instead of
habit. However, as Rogers[16] states, when manual dexterity is acclaimed to
the detriment of intellectual skill, such values are equally destructive of
those who hold them and those who are exposed to them.

Teachers should be clear on the difference between skills and habits. The
possession of skills is not merely the possession of habits. A habit is performed automatically with no self-criticism involved. Habits are acquired by
drill. In contrast, skills require the use of intelligent capacities. Skills are
acquired through training, which develops intelligence. Drill dispenses with
intelligence; training develops it. When Bruner[17] describes this process, he
states that the skilled performance that emerges may never be the same on
any two occasions. What is learned is competence, not particular performances. In learning for the professions, skills should not be routine. Instead,
one performance should be modified by its predecessors. In fact, the performance of a graduate student in nursing should focus on the discovery of
improved ways of performing.

In the clinical laboratory students should be faced with an element of the
unknown. Students attempt tasks that they have not accomplished yet, but
are no longer incapable of accomplishing. They are provided the opportunity
to apply knowledge to a variety of situations, using materials that they have
not encountered yet. The emphasis should be on the understanding of the
principles of practice instead of on mastery of a habitual performance. The
application of principles should be experimented with in a variety of situations leading to competency.

For example, in learning to administer an intramuscular injection the
student understands the principles of asepsis, anatomy, physiology, physics,
and pharmacology. The various types of equipment that might be used have
been manipulated in the college laboratory. So much is known about the
performance of the skill. At the same time what this student is ready to
learn, but is uncertain about, is how to select a site on the frail, aged, or
emaciated person versus the robust athlete or obese person; the needle to

use for children versus adults; and the position to use in the well-nourished, ambulatory person versus the person in pain and confined to bed. Such are the elements of learning to give an intramuscular injection that are best learned in a real-life situation.

Clinical laboratory practice, then, should have as its goal the engagement of the learner in activities for the purpose of acquiring competence both in the practice of motor skills and the development of the intellectual skills of synthesis, application, and evaluation. Yet this balance is not always achieved in clinical laboratory activities. Dewey[18] summarizes so aptly what professionals realize so fully, "that there is in general accord with the principle of habit, a tendency for every distinctive vocation to become too dominant, too exclusive and absorbing in its specialized aspect." The result is emphasis on skill or technical method at the expense of meaning. Educators must safeguard against this danger. The responsibilities of professionals are too weighty and the knowledge and skills of a profession too complex to reduce the acquisition to a process apart from thinking.

The clinical laboratory in undergraduate professional programs can provide a student with the opportunity to develop a foundation of skills based on knowledge by offering the opportunity to learn certain *essentials* in skills. Scheffler[19] ascribes three levels to skills; competence, proficiency, and mastery. He claims that knowing how to do something is one thing; knowing how to do it well is another; doing it brilliantly is still a third, which lies beyond the scope of know-how. Scheffler believes that we cannot hope to bring students to a high level of skill. As teachers, we all need to be reminded periodically that we should be "aware of the direction in which greatness lies, and teachers need to give students an analogous awareness even though they cannot train them to the point of greatness."[19] Basic professional training should be aimed toward the preparation of a student at the level of competence in an area of practice. Undergraduate students are basically setting out to acquire the "tools of the trade"—the knowledge and skills of the field of practice—what the practitioner already knows. The graduate student's activities should be quite different and aim to test theories and practices not commonly known to practitioners, that is, to discover new uses of theory and to formulate improved modes of nursing practice. Continual reminders of this concept are needed when expectations of both levels of students in the clinical laboratory are set. For example, while the undergraduate student learns to do health teaching for the newly diagnosed diabetic, the graduate student searches for the appropriate theories; that is, motivation theory, adult learning theory, to test strategies to improve adherence.

Finally, on the subject of skill learning, it is necessary to consider the length of the clinical laboratory sessions that would provide for optimal learning. The literature on skill learning advocates that a series of short practice sessions is more efficient than the same amount of practice in one continuous session. Smith and Smith[20] demonstrate that this rule has been valid for the sort of rote verbal learning used in laboratory experiments as well as for the learning of motor skills. However, the optimal interval between practice sessions has varied from one experiment to another. Experiments that favored massed practice over short sessions practice were those sessions that required a "warm-up," in which efficiency in tasks was important and rapidity was desired. Such characteristics should not be the objective of undergraduate clinical laboratory activities. Rapidity and repetitiveness are not valid objectives. Rogers[21] summarizes this concept so aptly when she states that the development of professional skills, whether of the hands or of the mind, is a lifetime process and will not ensue from extensive hours in a service setting spent in developing procedural dexterity.

Unlike the situation with the acquisition of knowledge, one cannot determine at what moment someone learned a skill. It is sensible to ask when one learned a fact; it is not sensible to ask when one learned a skill. One cannot be partly appraised of knowledge; one can be partly trained in a skill. This component of skill learning has numerous implications for the evaluation of clinical practice.

When a student is attempting to learn complex tasks, it has been found that it is more efficient in time, and advantageous to learning, to practice the parts first, free from the interference of coping with the real situation. The college laboratory, properly equipped as a simulated setting, provides the best opportunity for students to learn the parts. After the parts have been learned, the task in the clinical laboratory is to assimilate these parts.

In nursing education, all motor and intellectual skills that can be acquired apart from patients in the clinical setting should be learned in the college laboratory. The college laboratory should provide a wide use of audiovisual materials that may be used individually or in small groups by students at their own convenience and at their own pace. Many activities that formerly required a student's presence in the laboratory or classroom can now be provided through the use of technological devices. The student is thus provided with the freedom to practice the component parts of a task while taking the time needed to investigate, discover, make errors, and correct those errors. Simulated clinical laboratories should be arranged by faculty whenever possible. Through these means, the student can begin to combine component parts of a task in the relatively tension-free environment.

The amount of time that students should spend in the clinical laboratory has been the subject of much debate among nurse educators. It should be kept in mind that when a clinical laboratory is scheduled for a determined amount of time, it will prove to be insufficient for some students and unnecessarily long for other students to acquire a particular skill. Individuation of activities and time is needed. The length of time spent in a laboratory is no guarantee of the amount of learning that takes place. Students should be guided to determine for themselves how much time they need to learn a skill.

If it is not habit but skill that is the objective of the activities in the educational programs in nursing, then repetition of tasks is not necessary. This concept is also indirectly related to the question of time and the use of time. It is not necessary for a student to bathe each patient he is working with, make beds in every clinical laboratory period, or give all medications prescribed for that person. Once an objective is accomplished and a skill learned, it need not be repeated. Time should be used for acquiring new learnings. Teaching "how," which is directed at skill acquisition, is distinguished from teaching "to," which is directed at norm acquisition. To spend valuable laboratory time expanding the scope of the former at the expense of the latter is often a way of evading responsibility for those norms of action toward which teaching should in fact be directed.

Nurse educators readily admit that students of nursing must possess and apply knowledge and understanding to skill. But do these educators really provide for this type of learning? Is not the accuracy and efficiency of the practice of the skill often emphasized so much as to overshadow the importance of the acquisition and application of knowledge? And is a significant amount of time actually allowed for the acquisition and application of knowledge? Not if the practice of skills is expected before or too soon after theory to be applied to practice has been introduced. Not if time schedules are rigidly adhered to. Not if skills are first practiced in tense, demanding situations.

In the clinical laboratory, then, a nursing student performing a catheterization in that setting for the first time would be permitted to assemble equipment, determine the principles of aseptic technique, and prepare the client at his own pace. The client situation should not be a highly uncomfortable one or one that demands that the procedure be performed swiftly. Having removed the stresses of time, the focus of the student would then truly shift to the accuracy and knowledges to be brought to bear on the procedure. This use of time would also shift from the repetition of learned activities to the leisurely pursuit of new activities.

Psychomotor skill learning is a highly complex undertaking. It is of critical importance to a field like nursing. Nurse faculty need to explore the facets of skill learning and apply as many of the theories underlying the acquisition of skills as is possible. Attention to these matters can serve to greatly enhance teaching in nursing programs.

Encouragement of Critical Thinking

Clinical laboratory activities in the professions should train the learner to perform critically. The development of the ability to think critically demands that the learner be permitted to detect lapses in one's own knowledge and skill, correct them, profit from them, and therby improve practice. Scheffler believes that in professional education there must be room for training opportunities that will provide for the genuine exercise of students' judgment, as well as for critical reflection on the outcomes and strategic principles of such judgment. To achieve this the student must be given the opportunity to try different alternatives.

To plan for learning activities that are conducive to the development of critical thinking, the teacher needs a clear understanding of the terms. Critical thinking has been defined in a number of ways. Ennis[22] says that "critical thinking is the correct assessing of statements." Scheffler[23] claims that we talk of giving students the "ability to think critically" when we really want them "to acquire the habits and norms of critical thought." Gezi and Hadley[24] use the term "critical thinking" to refer broadly to the process that takes place in a problem-solving situation. In other words, problem solving refers to the situation in which critical thinking takes place. Inherent in these three selected definitions is the provision of opportunity for a student to learn the process of judging the worth of a knowledge, the effects of individual practice, and to develop the foresight to make the changes needed for improvement.

To promote critical thinking on the part of the student in the clinical laboratory, the teacher must provide an environment that is permissive so that the student is free from anxiety and feelings of inadequacy. A highly structured activity or a judgmental atmosphere defeats the purpose of the laboratory. Gezi and Hadley also suggest that the teacher be aware that the student needs knowledge to use as a base for his speculation. In addition to the knowledge base, the teacher may also need to point out events that are related and give cues as well as raise questions to help the student find other alternative modes of action.

Although most educators verbally subscribe to encouraging critical thinking in the learner, the identification of and implementation of the use of such strategies of teaching appear to be negligible. This is especially true of teaching in the clinical laboratory. In all fairness to these educators the problem may be rooted in a lack of investigation into the nature of critical thinking instead of an unwillingness to teach in this manner.

Phenix[25] explains that the method of teaching for any discipline is simply to provide experiences that encourage the student to engage actively in inquiry according to the patterns of discovery and validation characteristic of the discipline being studied. He advocates a spirit of inquiry that promotes critical thinking. Scheffler concurs by stating that teachers often aim at the achievement of certain sorts of learning in students here and now instead of at the development of a theoretical apparatus for explaining such learning and adapting their practice in the future. Rote learning prepares for today; critical thinking prepares for future practice. He contrasts *telling to,* which is aimed at securing immediate compliance, with *teaching to,* which is aimed at developing stable and general patterns of action. Such is the nature of critical thinking. More specifically, how can it be achieved?

Nursing students should be learning to test means to provide optimal personal hygienic care and comfort to the person who is terminally ill and not on rote learning of the steps involved in giving a bed bath. They should be learning about optimal dietary patterns and exercise programs aimed at preventing the occurrence or recurrence of a myocardial infarction, as opposed to spending much time on "how to make a bed" or "how to feed a patient." Change is about the only thing of which we can be certain. Rote tasks for the here and now will quickly render a professional obsolete.

The major fault of practice in the clinical laboratory in nursing education has often been that it is an anxiety-producing situation for students. Responsibilities surrounding the life and death of an individual are placed in their hands. Often, the student's knowledge about the health problem at hand, the equipment being used, and even the problem-solving process is sketchy. Obviously, this type of situation is not conducive to critical thinking. In such a situation the student is only interested in being told what to do in order to provide safe care during the crisis. Remove these responsibilities, and the performance of the student will change. Plan for students to participate in circumscribed activities related to health problems that they know well. Allow students to work only with equipment that has been manipulated in the college laboratory. Be sure that the problem-solving approach has been learned. Then raise questions. In this way habits of critical thought are more likely to develop.

Nurse educators should allow beginning students to learn to practice leisurely. Instead of holding them accountable for the care of patients, hold them accountable for learning. Use expert pratitioners for the care of patients. Remove from students the fear of endangering the life of an individual, and they are more likely to analyze what they are learning. Thus, they are more likely to acquire the habits of critical thought and apply what they have learned to future situations that are beyond the scope of their imagination at the present time.

Opportunity for Problem Solving

The clinical laboratory should provide the opportunity for students to engage in activities that require the finding of solutions to problems. The clinical laboratory is the place where the student brings to bear knowledge and skills in the solution of problems of the variety likely to be encountered in the profession. The problem-solving process involves defining the problem, collecting and analyzing pertinent data, hypothesizing consequences, testing hunches, and appraising the results. As Lindsey et al.[26] stated, the opportunity to test the meaning of key concepts through the use of the problem-solving process can be argued to be the heart of or the central purpose of the student's participation in the laboratory experience. Bruner,[27] in turn, writes that good "problems" are the chief vehicle for good curricula, whether one is in a classroom or alone in a cubicle with a teaching machine, whether one is working on "think" problems or laboratory exercises. In the clinical laboratory students have the advantage of actively testing their own proposed solutions and evaluating the results. The learner participates in an activity until the desired results are realized.

Closely related to the process of problem solving is that of analytical thinking. Dewey[28] discusses thinking as the accurate and deliberate instituting of connections between what is done and its consequences. Problem solving stimulates and implies thinking. Students actually learn to avoid errors if they have learned to think clearly and anticipate the results of their actions.

Activities undertaken by the learner in the clinical laboratory should present some optimal level of uncertainty. A persuasive argument is that uncertainty stimulates curiosity. Although these statements are widely accepted, Bruner cautions that activities that are too uncertain may arouse confusion and anxiety, with the effect of reducing exploration. Routine tasks also provoke little exploration and curiosity on the part of the student. It would seem that the task of the teacher is to assure that the student possesses the needed knowledge with which to approach an activity, but not the formulas for action. For example, a faculty member who delineates with the student major points to be included in discharge planning for a client leaves little opportunity for creative thinking, individualization of care, and problem solving. However, if that faculty member allows a student to assess that client and family situation and identify existing resources, cultural preferences, and past practices, the problem becomes what the most effective plan will be to raise this person to a higher level of wellness.

To solve problems, learners must be able to recall relevant principles that have been learned. They must be able to go beyond the knowledge at their command. Knowledge of facts, together with a basic understanding of the relationship between them, is a necessary prerequisite. To act without such knowledge is dangerous.

The factor of repetition appears to have no part to play in problem solving, except that it may be involved in the recall of subordinate principles. Studies have shown that "Once problem solution is achieved, learning appears to be unaffected by repetition. What is learned is highly resistant to forgetting."[29] The steps in problem solving do not require exactly matching performances or memorization. In fact, each laboratory session should provide new or different experiences or, at the very least, should provide some new knowledge, understanding, or satisfaction for the student if it is to be considered a satisfactory activity and legitimate use of time. Practice of the problem-solving process is valuable. The more practice students have, the better their ability to make generalizations that can be applied to other tasks encountered. However, practice in the same task is unwarranted. Repetition of the problem-solving process differs widely from the repetition of tasks. The problem-solving process should be applied to a variety of tasks. Hence, the expectation that all students should make beds and give baths in every lab session not only becomes a questionable use of time of the learner, but detracts from opportunities to work on solutions to new problems.

Although nurse educators readily verbalize the need for problem-solving activities for students in the clinical laboratory, the strategies used to provide for such activities often defeat the purpose. Nursing students must know and understand the problem-solving method thoroughly before entering the clinical laboratory. They must have tried and tested the method repeatedly in the college laboratory. They must also know and understand well all the principles to be applied to a skill performance before attempting it. This is not to say, however, that the learner must know precisely the steps involved in performing the skill. The knowledge needed to perform the skill must have been acquired; the problem-solving process should be mastered. However, the steps to be taken to apply that knowledge and process to the skill must not be prescribed, but instead should be discovered by the student.

However, this concept does not imply that students should be expected to apply the problem-solving technique to unexpected occurrences that may arise in the clinical laboratory unless they have already learned all of the principles that have to be applied to expected situations. Acting with too much uncertainty is not only undesirable, but unsafe.

To illustrate, suppose that a student has learned to provide certain aspects of care for a person who has suffered a myocardial infarction. The student is in the clinical laboratory to provide for the client's nutritional needs, progressive activity, and emotional support. If this person experiences a cardiac arrest, the expert practitioners should and must intervene and assume responsibility for all aspects of resuscitation and subsequent care. Because the student was not prepared for resuscitative measures, the most that he would be expected to do would be to observe the highly skilled techniques and the teamwork involved. To involve the student otherwise would be detrimental to learning and a personally traumatic experience that could lead to feelings of insecurity in the future. It would also be detrimental to the welfare of the client.

The problem-solving process is practiced especially well in determining how to assist a person to improvise in the home and work situation to satisfy health needs. How does one proceed without the assistance of sophisticated equipment? If the student knows the process of how to attack a problem, as well as the principles involved, he can help the client and the family discover that a seemingly impossible situation can become quite manageable. The student should be permitted to pursue this without clues from the teacher.

Opportunity for Observation

There should be an emphasis on observation as well as practice in professional laboratory activities. This emphasis should include learning how to observe, what to observe, how to record observations, and ultimately how to use the data collected in practice. In other words, the process of observation needs to be learned and practiced, initially apart from caring. The clinical laboratory is replete with opportunities for students to make accurate, orderly observations. Opportunity for the student to observe should, of course, precede practice sessions in any particular area of learning. A prerequisite to performing an observation is knowing the skills of observation. The skills of observation involve some very precise intellectual operations. The skills must be taught systematically.

Bruner[30] writes about observation as the heart of problem solving in the determination of a value. However, he also goes on to say that "looking with a highly assisted eye turns out to be central." An artist sees more in a painting than a casual observer untrained in the arts does. An expert practitioner of medicine notes more useful data in greeting a patient than one not trained in a medical specialty. Students must know "what" they are looking for and "how" to look before the process of observation becomes meaningful and fruitful to them. The "what" is the knowledge of the type of problem at hand. The "how" is the skill of making an observation.

During the period of observation, the student collects data. It is imperative for the learner to master this step in the problem-solving process before being expected to make decisions or professional judgments. The observation period is for the purpose, then, of student learning and should not be complicated with the responsibility of the student to render a service at the same time. Learners should be taught to concentrate on what actually happens with a view toward hypothesizing what factors could make it happen better the next time. The setting of limits, such as time limits, could also serve to interfere with the learning process. Students should be instructed to take as long as necessary to observe a situation as well as to compare as many similar situations as necessary to draw conclusions.

Another important aspect of the process of observation is the recording of data for later review and scrutiny. Clinical laboratory activities should involve the allowance of time for the accurate and useful recording of observations and impressions. Systematic recording in the clinical setting at the time the observations are made would lead to greater accuracy of interpretation and study at a later time, regardless of whether this study was to take place individually or in groups. Also, a record for periodic review would permit the student to apply facts and inferences to new situations at a later date.

Observation is a crucial element of the assessment phase of the nursing process. Knowledge on the part of the observer as to how to observe and what he is observing is equally crucial. A nursing student is hampered in making nursing judgments concerning a circulatory problem if there is no prior knowledge about the various circulatory problems, their similarities and differences, and their effect on the individual suffering from them. Hence, to require a student to observe in a clinical setting very early in a course before being allowed the time to acquire the basic knowledges is useless. Equally useless is the expectation that a student can make an observation before knowing what it is that constitutes the process of observation.

Also, the time for observations to be made in the clinical laboratory by nursing students need not be limited to weekdays between 7 a.m. and 3 p.m. The teacher merely needs to point out the availability and specific situations that would be likely to be meaningful to the learner; students then should be free to select from these situations ones of interest to them and observe them at any time and on any day that is right for them. In fact, an observation, such as that of the behavior of a person, can actually be enhanced by comparing findings at varied hours and at varied times throughout the week. So the consistent pattern of setting rigid laboratory hours each week can actually reduce the number of opportunities for the student to make useful observations.

Opportunity for Experimentation

The clinical laboratory is a place for the student to seek, to analyze, to select, and to use knowledge. The undergraduate does this in relation to existing knowledge, the graduate student experiments to discover new knowledge. This active participation by the learner facilitates learning through experimentation. The learner sees himself as an investigator. Lindsey writes that the laboratory must be a place where the learner does more than copy and perfect someone else's practice. The laboratory, instead, causes a student to analyze the practice of others in light of his knowledge and to develop a rewarding personal style of practice. It helps him to gain control of modes of inquiry appropriate to continued study of his behavior. Once again, the process is of central importance; a process that serves the practitioner throughout the span of a career.

The student, at the undergraduate level, should be allowed to test theories, add to present or existing knowledge, and reach predetermined solutions. This differs from the graduate level at which new theories and solutions are expected to be formulated. Bruner describes two interacting considerations in exploration; a sense of the goal of the task, and a knowledge of the relevance of tested alternatives to the achievement of that goal. The testing of alternatives yields information as to where one stands with respect to it. "Put in briefest form, direction depends upon knowledge of the results of one's tests, and instruction should have an edge over 'spontaneous' learning in providing more of such knowledge[31]." By providing structure in the laboratory activities and setting the conditions for learning, while at the same time allowing the student the freedom to put things together for himself, the teacher facilitates the production of autonomous thinkers. A precarious balance must be maintained between structured learning situations and freedom to learn within those limits. Nursing education has been notorious, for whatever reasons, for providing too much structure and too little freedom to students.

Discovery learning is an important aspect of learning through experimentation in clinical laboratory activities. Discovery learning is the very essence of the whole process of experimentation; it is the end point or product of experimentation. Discovery is defined as follows:

> . . . discovery, whether by a schoolboy going it on his own or by a scientist cultivating the growing edge of his field, is in its essence a matter of rearranging or transforming evidence in such a way that one is enabled to go beyond the evidence so reassembled to new insights.[32]

Emphasis on discovery helps the student to go about learning the very task of learning. To learn how to learn is the most valuable and lasting outcome of any educational system. Discovery is the *final step* in a sequence of learning; prerequisite knowledges must have preceded it. Discovery learning is based on knowledge. Gagné cautions that "the discovery method" is liable to gross misinterpretation in practical learning situations. He relates that some teachers have treated it as though it could be achieved with a minimum of instructions and prerequisite knowledge of principles and claims that this is obviously an incorrect point of view. Without prerequisite knowledge, no learning or inaccurate learning results.

The learner in the clinical laboratory can discover through a variety of situations structured by the teacher. Discovery may occur through personal inquiry, independent study, or group inquiry. Whatever the situation, the process is the same, namely freedom, that is, freedom of time and limits. Some activities may even lead to unproductive solutions. Friedlander claims that even this eventuality is all right. But students carry the responsibility to determine why they were unproductive. Teachers simply must allow students to be their own critics.

The clinical laboratory activities, to allow for discovery by students, must focus on fundamental ideas while judiciously sampling the detail on which to develop these ideas. The right activities in the right amount must be sampled. To accomplish this aim, these activities must span time and various subjects. Careful consideration of these few points by nurse educators would not only serve to enhance learning, but would free the teacher from some self-imposed constraints. Not all students need to care for the same circumscribed sets of clients or perform all psychomotor skills taught in a course. Instead, teaching by concept such as loss of patency, allows choices of clients with various problems with patency across the age spectrum. Some may care for a tracheostomy opening and others for a temporary colostomy opening.

The clinical laboratory in nursing education provides students with opportunities to develop skill in making accurate, orderly observations. Often the tendency of nurse educators is to provide students with activities that result in only a pseudo form of experimentation. Limits often are placed on time and the procedure. Directions are specific and little is left for the student to discover. These "cookbook" exercises provide no questions or uncertainty in the mind of the student. They know the answers before they begin. The result is no real participation in the development of solutions. In some instances, the student may possess inadequate knowledge and understanding of the situation and be unable to develop solutions. Both extremes are to be avoided. Instead, nursing students in the clinical laboratory should be well grounded in knowledge and should be allowed to solve problems and arrive at their own conclusions. After repeated attempts, the learner may well conclude that there are a number of acceptable or workable alternatives that can be selected to solve or alleviate a particular problem.

To expect a nursing student to observe and determine how to handle a frightened, withdrawn hospitalized child without having had the opportunity to learn basic related psychologic concepts, principles of the growth and development of the child, and knowledge of the anticipated reactions of the hospitalized child is irresponsible teaching. However, to set the above expectation after the student has acquired these prerequisite knowledges and is permitted the freedom to test a number of possible alternatives and record and systematically evaluate the resultant behaviors of the child is desirable teaching. Discovery learning and a spirit of inquiry are likely to result in the student exposed to the latter situation. Also, the student can be expected to develop an excitement and curiosity for learning that extends to subsequent practice.

Likewise, to expect nursing students to approach the clinical laboratory with a plan for precisely what is to be done instead of with a plan for what is to be learned is to preclude experimentation. Students should know what they are looking for, principles on which actions should be based, and alternative forms of action based on these principles. Students equipped with questions, hoping to answer them through experimenting with tried and tested alternatives, is the basis for laboratory activities. A different approach should be structured for different activities. The same approach to all activities will, in itself, reduce the possibility of experimentation and produce a practitioner dependent on others for direction.

Development of Professional Judgment

Participation in clinical laboratories in the professions requires that students be provided with the opportunity to develop professional judgment. Vocalis and Sheriff[33] identify three broad areas in which the student should develop increasing competence in the professional laboratory. One of these areas is professional responsibility. The use of sound professional judgment is an inherent part of the responsibility of any professional person. The clinical laboratory is rich in situations that provide the opportunity for learning the skill of judgment or decision making.

It follows that if students are expected to develop the ability to take a rational approach to decision making, then they should, during the program of study, be given the opportunity to learn to make professional decisions in selected situations. A laboratory situation can and should provide the conditions that facilitate these kinds of experience for students. The unexpected occurrences in the real setting are valuable opportunities for the student to develop competence in professional judgment *if* that student possesses the numerous knowledges needed to arrive at a valid judgment.

The professional practitioner is expected to be a person of knowledge. Phenix describes that person as highly skilled, but also one who acts with comprehension of the meaning of his actions. Such a person is prepared to deal with the complex situations that face the professional practitioner. As with each of the other elements, professional judgment requires that the individual have knowledge on which to base decisions and consequent actions. Knowing the process of decision making and accepting full responsibility for the consequences of one's actions is basic to professionalism. The clinical laboratory provides the opportunity for such learning, but the teacher should avoid placing on the student the responsibility of carrying out actions flowing from judgments until such a time as there is demonstrated readiness to assume this responsibility. Throughout the educational program the student is a learner and not a practitioner. Too heavy a responsibility too soon is overwhelming and serves to stifle learning of how to make sound professional judgments.

In nursing education, therefore, the student preparing to be a professional practitioner should be provided with the opportunity to learn to make judgments under guidance. However, it cannot be stressed enough that to learn to make judgments and to be responsible for making these judgments are two different matters. The former activity, "learning to," carries with it no responsibility. A skilled practitioner of nursing has this responsibility. The student is free to consult, test, and judge, but in early stages of course work is not required to carry out the actions that normally flow from judgments.

The "learning to" activities are appropriate early in the program of study. The responsibility for actually making judgments should be reserved until much later in the program of study, perhaps during the last year or even the last semester, when the knowledge needed to make that judgment has been acquired. This is an integrative activity in which responsibility is inherent; however, different students will be ready to assume this responsibility at different points in the program of study. To place such responsibility on a student too soon is likely to result in overcautiousness, dependence on direction to act, and lack of willingness to make independent judgments. The "safe" way to do it is resorted to quite often. To never expect responsible action may result in equally dependent behavior. It would result, at the very least, in an initial reluctance to make decisions.

To illustrate, consider once again the situation of the student caring for the person who experiences a cardiac arrest. To expect the student to participate in the resuscitative efforts for that person before having been afforded the opportunity to learn precisely what has occurred, what physical and chemical changes have resulted in the body, and what should be done to reverse the process is to place too much responsibility on the student at that time. Under such pressure, a learner's concerns and actions will likely revert to a compliance to the directions of others. Feelings of insecurity about making safe judgments are likely to be carried over in still other situations. Learning how to behave as a professional person and learning how to make independent judgments are obviously impeded. If the student is not prepared to handle that situation the only alternative is to remove the student from the situation. Without prior understanding of what occurs to a person experiencing a cardiac arrest, even observation of others rendering care is of limited value. If, on the other hand, the student is a senior who is competent in the knowledge and skills needed, participation in the resuscitative activities would prove to be meaningful to the student. Making rapid, valid judgments would be a source of much satisfaction and lasting learning for the knowledgeable, skillful student. Students need to be quite clear on when they are to plunge in and learn to make judgments, and when they are to withdraw and allow staff members to give expert and immediate care.

Encouragement of Creative Abilities

Clinical laboratory activities should be planned to elicit the creative abilities of the people involved. The learner must be encouraged to view and work with the problems at hand in his or her own manner. Dewey has written:

> . . . the first stage of contact with any new material, at whatever age of maturity, must be of the trial and error sort. An individual must actually try, in play or work, to do something with material in carrying out his own impulsive activity, and then note the interaction of his energy and that of the materials employed.[34]

Learners need to be allowed to try, to stumble, and yes, to fall while discovering their own method of proceeding, instead of being expected to mimic the actions of others. To allow for the trial and error described here, the student should not be entrusted with the responsibility for the service to the client until having judged his own actions to be correct. These actions should first be tested in the college laboratory. In the clinical laboratory further testing is done. Value judgments are made as to right or wrong, effective and ineffective, by the learner under the guidance of the teacher; however, the teacher must expect and allow for errors while learning. Only in such an atmosphere will inventiveness and self-expresssion result.

To be creative in the clinical laboratory, the nursing student must be assured that freedom of exploration and the freedom of expression are encouraged and rewarded by the system. The hands and minds of the learner must feel free to engage in creative activity, that is, to go beyond what has been learned. Of course, the kind and extent of guidance required will differ according to the individual student. But the time and place selected for clinical laboratory activities should also be unrestricted. Hours and setting rigidly determined should not be restrictive to the learner's creativity because of the demands for service in a particular set of circumstances. The educational needs of the learner must *always* supersede the service needs of the setting. Clients in a hospital may need much care during the morning hours. But student concerns are for learning and not for caring. Therefore, they do not necessarily learn in the morning and do not have to be in a hospital in the morning. At some levels in the curriculum, the morning hours may be undesirable due to the hecticness of the situation.

The teacher is responsible for setting the stage or atmosphere for creative learning. Students are responsible for using their creative abilities to learn. However, as Phenix has so aptly stated, the teacher must exemplify an imaginative quality of mind. The teacher might well serve as the model of a creative mind. This creativity manifests itself in the teaching, practice, and scholarly pursuits of the faculty member.

Nursing students are to be prepared for practice in an educational program that provides for individual and changing approaches to the application of knowledge. Such an approach is intended to mold a practitioner that will be continually striving to find improved ways of rendering nursing care to people throughout their practice career. Freedom of exploration and expression in the clinical laboratory is needed. To accomplish this aim, a nursing student requires freedom from the restrictions of time and the responsibility of rendering "total care" to an assigned number of clients. Under such a regimen, students are likely to succumb to pressures and resort to following standard procedures. Creativity is thereby stifled.

Nurse faculty need to train themselves to be models of a creative mind. This is no easy task because most faculty are not themselves products of educational programs that encouraged them to be creative. Hence, faculty have the dual responsibility of developing this mode of thinking and behaving in themselves as well as determining how to inculcate such values and aspirations in their students.

To be assigned to give total care to a client experiencing respiratory distress in order to learn about difficulties in respiration and the nursing interventions needed is narrow and restrictive of such learning. Too little time will be spent on the central objective. Too much time will be spent tending to the hygienic needs of this person as well as other aspects of care needed. Instead, the student might be allowed the freedom to interact with five or six persons experiencing respiratory distress to compare respiratory patterns, observable symptomology, and limitations on activities of daily living. Also, this student could investigate the technologic and chemotherapeutic agents used to relieve respiratory distress and formulate plans of care for a variety of clients. Such an exercise could be performed in an agency setting, a home setting, or both. Creative ways to provide comfort, relieve distress, and improve the client's quality of living would be more likely to result.

When the objective is to learn to irrigate a colostomy, the student's time in the clinical laboratory should be spent solely on the problems involved in performing successful irrigation. An identification of the similarities and differences of problems of persons who have a colostomy should be expected. Creative insights into use of equipment, positioning, dietary habits, and health teaching should be encouraged. To spend a day or more giving total care to a person with a colostomy should not be expected. In such a situation only a minute portion of time might be spent on the central objective. In fact, it might even be lost in a maze of other activities.

Provision for Transfer of Knowledge

Clinical laboratory activities should serve to facilitate the transfer of knowledge from one type of situation to another—from college laboratory to clinical laboratory. The clinical laboratory setting provides a fertile field for the student to encounter situations in which basic knowledge must be applied to a wide variety of problems in varying circumstances. Problems presented in the field can be analyzed in light of resultant experiences and provide the culmination of learning for the student. To facilitate this transfer of knowledge, Zasowska advocates that the laboratory experience parallel classroom instruction so that the learner recognizes a direct relationship between course content and laboratory activity. Studies have demonstrated differences between teacher perceptions and student perceptions of factors assisting knowledge application in the clinical laboratory.[35,36]

Bruner has written that the first object of any act of learning, beyond the pleasure it may give, is that it should serve us in the future. Clinical laboratory provides the opportunity for the student to apply previously learned principles to "real" or practical situations such as will be encountered in future practice. Real-life situations reveal to the student the needs and shortcomings in society. The student who is faced with such situations can put acquired knowledge to work in terms of alleviating the problems. These experiences also enable the learner to recognize more readily the need to respond to similar situations in the future. Caution must be exercised by the teacher to avoid emphasis on the present demands as a sacrifice for futuristic thinking.

In the clinical laboratory the learner is enabled to translate theory into practice by raising questions, stimulating creative thinking, and producing action. But the laboratory activities must be structured by the teacher to produce these outcomes. They cannot be left to chance. The motivation to transfer knowledge to actual situations is usually higher in the clinical laboratory than in the classroom. "All instruction," writes Bruner,[37] "consists of leading the learner through a sequence of statements and restatements of a body of knowledge that increase the learner's ability to grasp, transform, and transfer what he is learning." In speaking of motivation, McClelland contends that the more an individual can link the newly developed network to related actions, the more the change in both thought and action is likely to occur and endure. In the clinical laboratory, newly acquired knowledges take on new meaning for the student and become a guide in further action.

All professional students are anxious to be involved in the real action. This motivation should be capitalized on. Yet it should be done only when a readiness for transfer is demonstrated.

In the clinical laboratory in nursing education every opportunity is provided for the student to apply theory to practice as each individual determines it should be applied. For the faculty member to suggest methods, give directions, or refer a student to procedures makes this transfer of knowledge on the part of the student unnecessary. Guidance should be offered by the faculty member and provided when it is sought by the student. And this guidance should be in the form of questions and thought-provoking comments that will require the student to think through a situation, recall principles learned, and recognize a logical application of these principles to a situation. Cookbook responses on the part of the teacher tend to stifle, delay, or even destroy a student's ability to transfer knowledge from one client problem to another or from a simulated situation to the real situation.

Clinical laboratory activities should run concurrently with materials dealt with in theory in the classroom. Classroom demonstrations of skill-oriented activities are generally ineffective. However, recorded demonstrations for use in the college laboratory are desirable wherein students discover answers or methods on their own. The student should be allowed to apply theory to practice very soon after the theory is learned; otherwise, the ability to make the transfer is greatly diminished or lost. Also, the opportunity to transfer knowledge should be available in more than one setting in a given time. It is not enough to learn about the care of a person recovering from a myocardial infarction by observing him and relating to him solely in the hospital setting. It is essential that within this same period the application of principles should be made to such persons in the home and work settings. So, the opportunity to transfer knowledge extends beyond settings.

Also, the student must learn how to apply a principle to people in different age groups and at different levels of wellness. While a student is learning the effects of pressure on skin at various points in the body, numerous films, filmstrips, books, and articles related to the subject should be used to reinforce classroom discussions. Questions might be raised as to what occurs locally to the skin when prolonged pressure is applied. Questions might be raised as to how to prevent this occurrence or treat it once it has already occurred. Provision for observation of the effects of pressure on the skin of persons in various levels of wellness should be provided for as soon as the essential knowledges have been acquired by the student. Provision should also be made for the care of such persons when this learning is acquired and caring activities are appropriate. In the former instance, the teacher is continually playing the role of an advocate of learning. The student is always an active learner, a searcher of knowledge. The direct antithesis of this learning would be to enumerate major causes of pressure on the skin of a hospitalized person, describe the nursing care needed to relieve this pressure, and to care for a person with a decubitus.

Participation in Integrative Activities

Clinical laboratory activities are undertaken as integrative instead of initial learning activities. Integrative activities are the culmination of all the learning that has gone before. Rogers writes that college laboratories provide opportunity for students to develop beginning skills in application, testing, and affirming of theoretical content. The more complex tasks, as well as the synthesis and use of various knowledges and skills, are practiced in the clinical laboratory. Students who are placed in the clinical laboratory, then, are presumed to possess at least the basic knowledges and skills of their field of study.

> . . . a shift in emphasis from experiences as beginning points of learning to experiences as the end points of learning might avoid some of the unfortunate characteristics of teaching procedures which have in the past often focused exclusively on learning *by* experience—procedures in which experiences have been introduced in the hope of gaining other types of learning products, with the general result that many unwanted learning products (by-products) have also crept in . . . .[38]

The above ideas support the division of "whole" versus "part" learning. In learning complex tasks, then, it is usually advantageous to possess a sound knowledge base and then proceed to practice the component parts. Progression to the practice of the whole would follow. If the clinical laboratory is to provide for integrative activities, it would follow that the learning of the "parts" would more appropriately and efficiently be performed in the college laboratory, while the practice of the whole would be reserved for the clinical laboratory. In the college laboratory, the student is shielded from the pressures of the real situation. The desired learning can result. The unwanted learning is less likely to occur.

For example, in learning to do a health assessment, the student needs to know the anatomy and physiology of the body, normal versus abnormal appearance and functioning of each body system, and use of the various techniques and approaches used to examine the body. Knowledge of each of these three areas needs to be learned sequentially; skills related to examining the body need to be practiced separately in the college and then clinical laboratory, that is, conducting an examination of the eye, the ear, the abdomen, as an integrative activity, the student ultimately conducts a complete health assessment in a clinical setting.

Clinical laboratory activities serve to illustrate relationships to the student. In this setting, the link between knowledges is visualized by the student. This ability to see relationships is essential in the educative process for, as Dewey[39] has stated, experiences may be so disconnected from one another that, while each is agreeable or even exciting in itself, if they are not linked cumulatively to one another they generate dispersive, disintegrated habits. Such experiences are misleading. Yet links in knowledge cannot be made until separate knowledges have been acquired. The educator faces the task of using appropriately the physical and social surroundings in both the college and clinical laboratory to provide the opportunity for experiences that are meaningful and interrelated.

The clinical laboratory in nursing education provides a wealth of integrative activities for the learner. The determination that seems to be of major importance lies in when and how students should participate in these activities. Obviously, the nursing student should be allowed to participate in integrative activities such as planning for and administering many aspects of care to a client or family. But this should be attempted only after a maximum amount of knowledge and/or skill has been acquired and demonstrated in the college laboratory. The expectation that students participate in integrative activities should be restricted to the end of the program of study for most students. How soon a student proceeds to participate in such activities is a very individual matter and should be planned for and with each student.

Before caring for a client in a postoperative period, a student must, in general, know how to maintain a patent airway, monitor and interpret vital signs, maintain the sterility of a wound, and provide for the safety and comfort of that person. The knowledges and skills inherent in each of these aspects of care should be acquired in the classroom and study situations and be practiced in the college laboratory. The care of a person postoperatively in the clinical laboratory is a culminating activity for which one student may be ready soon after the above activities are introduced, and for which another student may require a much longer time to learn. But no student should care for a postoperative client until competence in each of the components of care has been demonstrated.

How often have students been assigned to give care to a patient when that student knows how to administer only a portion of that care? How often have students voiced concern to their instructors about an impending task that they feel they are not competent to perform? And how often have instructors said, "Let me know when you are ready to do that, and I'll help you. Or I'll demonstrate it to you"? Demonstrations have no place in the clinical laboratory. Demonstrations are done in the college laboratory. The faculty member does not render care in the clinical laboratory. The faculty member functions as a teacher and not a practitioner. The faculty member is there to give guidance to students and not to render care to clients. Students should not give care to clients unless they are completely knowledgeable about that care. Students should not be assigned to integrative activities if they have not learned the individual activities. No value can be derived from approaching an integrative task when the component parts have not been sufficiently understood to see relationships between the parts.

Utilization of the Team Concept

Clinical laboratory activities need to include a provision for inducting the learner into the team setting and preparing him to make maximum contributions as a team member. "Although the major emphasis in the curricula will quite likely focus on preparing the student to function confidently and competently as a sole responsible agent, his role as a member of a team working to provide a service cannot be excluded."[40] In the health professions, the team concept is growing in importance. Professionals must learn to work together to provide efficient and effective health services. An isolated type of practice is no longer effective. Also, in an age of specialization, the expertise of each team member is needed to render quality care.

The team concept will not be used fully if left to chance learning. Instead, the knowledge and skills of interacting with health team members should be provided within the context of professional programs of study. In the educational program the team concept must not only be discussed in theory, but emphasized in practice in the clinical laboratory activities. Students should have knowledge of the basic theories of the team concept as well as have a working knowledge of the other team members involved in providing a service. They should understand the contribution of each member toward that service. Knowledge of the various other professional or colleague relationships, as well as of the nonprofessional personnel, is essential.

The clinical laboratory provides the student with the opportunity to observe team concepts and, subsequently, with the opportunity to practice within the system of relationships. The study of the composition of the health team and the function, roles, and activities of the various members of the health team should proceed soon after the nursing student gains an image of self as a health care provider. Emphasis on the uniqueness of function of various health workers as well as overlap of activities among them is essential. Collaborative roles, leadership activities, and effective means of communication should be included *before* the student encounters other health team members in the clinical laboratory. The student should know how to handle and benefit from what is about to be encountered. Like knowledge of any other laboratory activity, it would be risky to leave it to chance.

Planned laboratory activities such as interdisciplinary conferences, referrals, and consultations should be a part of every nursing student's experience. These activities should be provided throughout the nursing courses so that learners come to view them as an integral part of their practice of nursing. Making "rounds" with health team members on a regular basis would be useful to planning care.

In fact, students can no longer learn about health team members and the health care delivery system in isolation. It is recommended that health professionals teach the theory and plan clinical laboratory activities jointly for their students. Interdisciplinary courses are advocated. It would be ideal to have the interdisciplinary approach to health care permeate the curricula of each school or department. An interdisciplinary endeavor in learning would provide the best model for interdisciplinary practice by students. Students must learn together if they are to be expected to practice together in joint activities rather than parallel activities.

The proper utilization of the team concept, both in preparation for and use of in the clinical setting, is a very demanding concept for faculty. Perhaps it is the most demanding of the fourteen essential elements. It requires that health professional faculty plan and teach together. Such team-teaching strategies are time consuming and sometimes even painful. It requires a "thrasing out" of the responsibilities and rights of each as a professional. In fact, it requires the highest level of collaboration. All of these demands are made on persons who themselves had no such preparation in their own educational programs. But their greatest asset is a knowledge of what the process should be and a vision of what the resultant service to society could be. Extreme patience and dedication are the added ingredients that are needed to accomplish the goal. If faculty achieve it, students are more likely to achieve it.

If the team concept, as described, was to be incorporated into health professional curricula, it is believed that a new and more effective generation of health practitioners would emerge from our schools.

Summary of Concepts Inherent in the Essential Elements

1. Client contact
   a. always involves contact with clients
   b. emphasizes how to apply knowledge to care
   c. type of contact determines time and place

2. Objectives
   a. clearly stated objectives for each laboratory session
   b. integral part of the course
   c. feedback provided on each objective
   d. laboratory activities contribute to goal achievement
3. Competent Guidance
   a. central activity of teacher is teaching
   b. carefully structure laboratory activities
   c. individualize clinical activities
   d. allow for self-correction and eventual self-sufficiency
4. Individuation
   a. consider needs, values, and goals of each student
   b. assist students to self-initiate and self-select activities
   c. time spent in laboratory varies among students
5. Psychomotor skill learning
   a. knowledge and understanding prerequisite
   b. avoid repetition and habit formation
   c. each performance modified by predecessors
   d. varying time intervals for acquisition of skills among learners
6. Critical thinking
   a. individual performs critically—detects lapses, corrects them, profits from them
   b. individual acquires the habits and norms of critical thought
7. Problem solving
   a. involves defining the problem, collecting and analyzing pertinent data, hypothesizing consequences, testing hunches, appraising results
   b. a level of uncertainty desirable
   c. students recall and use relevant principles
   d. repetition has no part to play in problem solving
8. Observation
   a. know the process of observation
   b. allow time for making observations
   c. no responsibility for care during initial observation periods
   d. allow time for recording observations and impressions
9. Experimentation
   a. involves testing of theories

      b. reach predetermined solutions

      c. add to existing knowledge

10. Professional judgment

      a. provide opportunities to develop professional judgments

      b. use decision-making processes

11. Creativity

      a. encourage freedom of exploration

      b. encourage freedom of expression

      c. allow for errors while learning

      d. reward for inventiveness and self-expression

12. Transfer of knowledge

      a. apply knowledge to varied situations

      b. translate theory into practice

13. Integrative activities

      a. component *part* learning precedes integrative activities

      b. culminating activities occur in clinical laboratory

      c. *caring* activities performed later in program of study

14. Team concept

      a. knowledge of team concept

      b. knowledge of other team members

      c. participation as a contributing team member

Implications of the Essential Elements for the Clinical Laboratory in Nursing Education

A close examination of the essential elements of the clinical laboratory as outlined reveals an endless number of implications for nurse educators. A consideration of the activities currently practiced in the clinical laboratory viewed in light of the essential elements serves as a point of departure for future planning in regard to this important aspect of the total curriculum. There are implications for two specific groups of teachers: (1) teachers of nursing in undergraduate programs, and (2) teachers of teachers being prepared in graduate programs.

    Teachers of nursing in undergraduate programs need to review their use of the clinical laboratory in their own teaching in light of the essential elements. Determining the direction in which change in teaching strategies should proceed would thus be more easily and accurately accomplished. Some suggestions follow.

First and foremost, faculty members who teach nursing would benefit from serious consideration of the idea that there is a difference between using knowledge and learning how to use knowledge. There is a difference between caring for clients and learning how to care for clients. Adequate knowledge gained in both classroom and laboratory settings about how to care is needed before investing students with the responsibility to give care. Learning is not synonymous with caring. Faculty are invested primarily with the responsibility for learning and not for caring.

The idea of students giving care to clients needs to be placed in proper perspective. Giving total care to clients is an integrative activity that, from an educational point of view, is an activity reserved until the latter part of the program of study, when the knowledges and skills of the various components of that care have been acquired. A careful determination of when, where, and how undergraduate students need to be taught a skill, and when, where, and how they need to be taught how to use that skill in a whole scheme seems to be essential.

Second, the quality and the orientation of the clinical laboratory activities of nursing students needs upgrading to make it a truly educational experience. Efficiency of time and learning must be scrutinized. Teachers must explore ways to use the essential elements of the laboratory concept *consistently* in the clinical laboratory. To use the concept occasionally, in some settings, or when it is convenient is not adequate. Perhaps once a true recognition of the deficiencies that exist are made, the variety of approaches that can be taken to correct these deficiencies will be more readily apparent.

Additionally, the traditional and confining method of assigning a client(s) to students for complete care must be relinquished. Students should be assigned to learning activities, not clients; clients need care and care implies responsibility. Freedom from the restrictions of providing safe care is needed by students. As Russell has warned, the concern for being "safe and proper" perpetuates outmoded and inadequate practices. Even licensing requirements exert an undue influence on local educational theory and practice. Rigid requirements of state boards of nursing must be abolished and superseded by quality standards set by education. Faculty members do not follow standards; faculty members set standards.

Finally, the long hours spent in the clinical laboratory and the small percentage of this time apparently used solely for learning imply that the clinical laboratory may not have to be used as extensively as it presently is. More freedom from the long hours spent each week in the clinical laboratory and more flexibility of time as well as settings and activities for each student would seem to free greatly the total curriculum for needed change. The telescoping of time spent in the clinical laboratory would permit time for other learning available on the campus. On the other extreme, though, dangerously few clinical hours have been set in some courses. Enough clinical practice time must be required to permit the development of competency in the typical student. Faculty must carefully determine, sometimes through trial and error, the amount of time needed on the average to accomplish a set of clinical laboratory objectives.

Nurse faculty state that the scarcity of clinical facilities near the campus and the clinical hours dictated by various sources impinge on change that might otherwise occur. Freedom from long-standing dedication to prescribed hours in the clinical laboratory would facilitate change and make available innumerable opportunities for more timely learning activities. Because it usually happens that most faculty compete for the same hours in clinical settings, a more flexible approach should reduce the problem of access and availability.

Teachers in graduate schools who are preparing teachers for undergraduate programs in nursing might place more emphasis on strategies of teaching in the clinical laboratory. Strategies for teaching in the classroom are routinely explored. Strategies for teaching in the clinical laboratory, the heart of professional education, have been less notable in course outlines. Perhaps increased opportunity for future teachers to apply theory to practice with guidance is also needed. Just as changes in the services of professional practitioners must start with the educational program of which they are a product, so changes in the type of teaching done by teachers at the senior college or university level must start with changes in the educational programs that prepare these teachers.

Suggestions for the Refinement
of the Use of the Laboratory in Nursing Education

The clinical laboratory activities as being practiced in undergraduate programs in nursing tend at the present to embody the essential elements of the laboratory concepts to varying extents. The inference is that to improve the use of the clinical laboratory in educational programs in nursing, nursing education must raise the basic question about what the clinical laboratory is about and what it is that students should do there. Answers to these questions, then, would lead to new advances in the use of the clinical laboratory in baccalaureate education in nursing. Let us take a forward look at what nursing education would be like.

Nurse educators would shift the focus of their responsibilities in their clinical teaching. They would redirect their energies from close and continual supervision to guidance aimed at independent action. The need for the teacher to be present in the clinical laboratory would be greatly reduced.

The teacher would instead use her time in preparing students for practice and in designing opportunities for the student to apply theory to practice. The teacher would guide instead of direct activities. Students would be assisted to learn instead of being directed as to what to do. The teacher would raise questions instead of answer questions. Creative behavior and critical thinking would be encouraged and rewarded. Divergent thinking would be valued.

Students, on the other hand, would participate to a much greater extent in planning for and selecting their clinical laboratory activities. Their individual needs, interests, and aptitude would be given priority consideration. Their clinical laboratory activities would not know the boundaries of time or setting. Students would learn *about* giving care before *giving* care. Theory would be learned and tested in the college laboratory before application in the clinical laboratory. Students would *learn to do* instead of *learn by doing*. Students would experience an excitement about learning the art and science of nursing that has been unmatched in the past.

Nursing education needs to prepare young practitioners who are seekers of knowledge and who are full of speculation and doubt, all in the interest of giving quality care. They need to question everything they see. They need to hypothesize better ways of doing things. To achieve this, the student must have the opportunity to accomplish an objective in an atmosphere of freedom. Nursing would be more likely to attract and retain the most able students with the greatest potential. They would be less likely to become disillusioned about nursing. Before acquiring prerequisite knowledges and skills for caring, the learner would be freed from the responsibility of rendering care to clients. Caring for clients would be a culminating activity reserved largely for the end of the educational program.

Administrators of educational programs in nursing would relinquish the control of the selection of clinical laboratory settings to faculty. Faculty would be permitted to select and use a wide variety of clinical laboratory settings in a particular area to accomplish their course objectives and satisfy the individual learning needs of students. Contractual agreements with community health agencies would need to provide for a fluidity of movement of the faculty and the students within the agency, as well as in and out of the agency. Time schedules and service expectations would be eliminated. Faculty would also be free to use nonagency-related resources in the community in concert with hospitals.

If the above suggestions were implemented, the use of the clinical laboratory in nursing education could begin to approximate more closely the use of the clinical laboratory in teacher education, medical education, and education for social work. The student of nursing would be provided with contact with the client in the clinical laboratory. However, the student would learn how to give a professional service without carrying the responsibility for actually rendering that service. Like other professional students, the nursing student would have the freedom to move in and out of situations instead of being tied to a particular setting for a fixed number of hours or weeks. After having acquired the intellectual and motor skills essential to giving nursing care, the student would be allowed the opportunity to render such care. Guidance instead of elbow supervision would be provided. In keeping with the educational practices of the other professions considered, nursing education would move in the direction of providing students with a higher quality and more efficient system of education.

Notes

1. Blair, L. C. *An exploration of the nature and function of laboratory experiences in the development of general education courses offered at State Teachers College, Indiana, Pennsylvania.* Unpublished doctoral dissertation, Teachers College, Columbia University, 1953, p. 33.

2. Rogers, M. *Educational revolution in nursing.* New York: The Macmillan Company, 1961, p. 37.

3. Bruner, J. The skill of relevance or the relevance of skills. *Saturday Review*, 1970, 53, April 18, 1970, p. 68.

4. Zasowska, M. A. *A descriptive survey of significant factors in the clinical laboratory experience in baccalaureate education for nursing.* Unpublished doctoral dissertation, Teachers College, Columbia University, 1967, p. 16.

5. Hanson, J. Learning by experience. In *Language and concepts in education.* Smith, B. O., & Ennis, R. H. (Ed.). Chicago: Rand McNally and Company, 1961, p. 7.

6. Stratemeyer, F. The professional sequence. In *Teacher education for a free people.* Cottrell, D. P. (Ed.). New York: The American Association of Colleges for Teacher Education, 1956, p. 73.

7. Lindsey, M. *Inquiry into teaching behavior of supervisors in teacher education laboratories.* New York: Teachers College Press, Teachers College, Columbia University, 1969, p. 24.

8. McClelland, D. C. Toward a theory of motive acquisition. *American Psychologist*, 1965, 20 (5), p. 329.

9. Bruner, J. *Toward a theory of instruction.* New York: W. W. Norton and Company, Inc., 1966, p. 53.

10. Gagné, R. M. *The conditions of learning.* New York: Holt, Rinehart & Winston, Inc., 1965, p. 163.

11. Blair, L. C. *An exploration of the nature and function of laboratory experiences in the development of general education courses offered at State Teachers College, Indiana, Pennsylvania.* Unpublished doctoral dissertation, Teachers College, Columbia University, 1953, p. 29.

12. Dewey, J. *Experience and education.* New York: The Macmillan Company, 1938, pp. 10–11.

13. Pellegrino, E. D. Human values and the medical curriculum. *Journal of the American Medical Association,* 1969, *209* (9), p. 1352.

14. Lindsey, M., et al. *Inquiry into teaching behavior of supervisors in teacher education laboratories.* New York: Teachers College Press, Teachers College, Columbia University, 1969, p. 17.

15. Ryle, G. *The concept of mind.* London: Hutchinson and Company, 1949, p. 29.

16. Rogers, M. E. *Educational revolution in nursing.* New York: The Macmillan Company, 1961, p. 60.

17. Bruner, J. The skill of relevance or the relevance of skills. *Saturday Review,* April 18, 1970, p. 67.

18. Dewey, J. *Democracy and education.* New York: The Macmillan Company, 1916, p. 360.

19. Scheffler, I. *Conditions of knowledge.* Chicago: Scott, Foresman and Company, 1965, p. 95.

20. Smith, K. V., & Smith, M. F. *Cybernetic principles of learning and educational design.* New York: Holt, Rinehart & Winston, Inc., 1966, p. 38.

21. Rogers, M. E. *Educational revolution in nursing.* New York: The Macmillan Company, 1961, p. 38.

22. Ennis, R. H. A concept of critical thinking. *Harvard Educational Review,* 1962, *32* (Winter), p. 83.

23. Scheffler, I. *The language of education.* Springfield, Illinois: Charles C. Thomas, 1960, p. 99.

24. Gezi, K., & Hadley, F. Strategies for developing critical thinking. *Journal of Nursing Education,* 1970, 9 (2), p. 10.

25. Phenix, P. H. *Realms of meaning.* New York: McGraw-Hill Book Company, 1964, p. 339.

26. Lindsey, M., et al. *Inquiry into teaching behavior of supervisors in teacher education laboratories.* New York: Teachers College Press, Teachers College, Columbia University, 1969, p. 4.

27. Bruner, J. The skill of relevance or the relevance of skills. *Saturday Review,* April 18, 1970, 53, p. 66.

28. Dewey, J. *Democracy and Education*. New York: The Macmillan Company, 1916, p. 177.
29. Gagné, R. M. *The conditions of learning*. New York: Holt, Rinehart & Winston, Inc., 1965, p. 163.
30. Bruner, J. The skill of relevance or the relevance of skills. *Saturday Review*, April 18, 1970, 53, p. 66.
31. Bruner, J. *Toward a theory of instruction*. New York: W. W. Norton and Company, Inc., 1966, p. 44.
32. Bruner, J. *On knowing*. Cambridge, Massachusetts: The Belknap Press of Harvard University Press, 1966, p. 82.
33. Vocalis, J., & Sheriff, M. *A study of prefessional laboratory experiences prior to student teaching in the pre-service program in childhood education at Teachers College, Columbia University*. Unpublished doctoral dissertaion, Teachers College, Columbia University, 1961, p. 8.
34. Dewey, J. *Democracy and education*. New York: The Macmillan Company, 1916, p. 181.
35. Olson, E. M. Baccalaureate students' perceptions of factors assisting knowledge application in the clinical laboratory. *Journal of Nursing Education*, 1983, 22 (1), p. 18–21.
36. Wang, A. M., & Blumberg, P. A study on interaction techniques of nursing faculty in the clinical area. *Journal of Nursing Education*, 1983, 22 (4), p. 144–151.
37. Bruner, J. *Toward a theory of instruction*. New York: W. W. Norton and Company, Inc., 1966, p. 49.
38. Hanson, J. Learning by experience. In *Language and concepts in education*. Smith, B. O., & Ennis, R. H. (Ed.). Chicago: Rand McNally and Company, 1961, p. 22.
39. Dewey, J. *Experience and education*. New York: The Macmillan Company, 1938, p. 14.
40. Lindsey, M., et al. *Inquiry into teaching behavior of supervisors in teacher education laboratories*. New York: Teachers College Press, Teachers College, Columbia University, 1969, p. 13.

Bibliography

Ausubel, D. P. Learning by discovery. *Educational Leadership*, 1962, 20 (2), 113, 117.
Banks, M. E. Alternative community placements for students. The challenge of day care centers. *Nursing and Health Care*, 1982, 3(4), 196–198,

Becktell, P. J. The effect of freedom on the learning of gifted nursing students. *Journal of Nursing Education*, 1981, *20*(9), 24–30.

Benner, P., & Wrubel, J. Skilled clinical knowledge: The value of perceptual awareness. *Nurse Educator,* 1982, *7*(3), 11–17.

Berggren, H., & Zagornik, A. D. Teaching nursing process to beginning students. *Nursing Outlook*, 1968, *16*(7), 32–35.

Bevil, C. W., & Gross, L. C. Assessing the adequacy of clinical learning settings. *Nursing Outlook*, 1981, *29*(11), 658–661.

Brown, B. J. Clinical excellence. *Nursing Administration Quarterly*, 1981, *6*(1), entire issue.

Brown, S. T. Faculty and student perceptions of effective clinical teachers. *Journal of Nursing Education*, 1981, *20*(9), 4–15.

Bruner, J. *On knowing.* Cambridge: The Belknap Press of Harvard University Press, 1966.

––––––. The act of discovery. *Harvard Educational Review*, 1961, *31* (Winter), 21–32.

––––––. *The process of education.* New York: Random House, 1960.

––––––. The skill of relevance or the relevance of skills. *Saturday Review*, April 18, 1970, *53*, 66–68.

––––––. *Toward a theory of instruction.* New York: W. W. Norton and Company, Inc., 1966.

Cantor, M. M., Schroeder, D. M., & Kurth, S. W. The experienced nurse and the new graduate: Do their learning needs differ? *Nurse Educator*, 1981, *6*(1), 17–22.

Chickadonz, G. H., Burke, M. M., Fitzgerald, S., & Osterweis, M. Development of a primary care setting for nursing education. *Nursing and Health Care*, 1982, *31*(2), 83–87, 92.

Congreve, W. J. *An experiment in independent learning.* Chicago: University of Chicago, 1963.

Cosper, B. Coping with an increased student–faculty ratio. *American Journal of Nursing*, 1976, *76*(10), 1642–1644.

Cotanch, P. H. Self-actualization and professional socialization of nursing students in the clinical laboratory experience. *Journal of Nursing Education*, 1981, *20*(8), 4–14.

Davidhizar, R. N. Helping students help themselves. *Nursing and Health Care*, 1982, *31*(3), 138–140.

Department of Baccalaureate and Higher Degree Programs. *Utilization of the clinical laboratory in baccalaureate nursing programs.* New York: National League for Nursing, 1978, Publication No. 15-1726.

DeLorey, P. E. Selecting learning experiences which encourage deviant behavior. *American Journal of Nursing*, 1969, *69*(4), 800–803.

deTornyay, R. *Strategies for teaching nursing.* New York: John Wiley & Sons, Inc., 1982.

————. The effect of an experimental teaching strategy on problem solving abilities of sophomore nursing students. *Nursing Research*, 1968, *17*(2), 108–114.

Dobbie, B. J., & Karlinsky, N. A self-directed clinical practicum. *Journal of Nursing Education*, 1982, *21*(9), 39–41.

Eble, K. E. *The craft of teaching*. San Francisco: Jossey–Bass Co., 1976.

Eliot, J. E. *Toward more effective teaching*. Publication of Western Council on Higher Education for Nursing, 1964, 7–63.

Ennis, R. H. A concept of critical thinking. *Harvard Educational Review*, 1962, *32* (Winter), 81–109.

Fitts, P. Factors in complex skill learning. *Training, Research, and Education*. Pittsburgh, Pennsylvania: University of Pittsburgh Press, 1962.

Fitts, P., & Posner, M. *Human performance*. Belmont, California: Brooks/Cole Publishing Co., 1967.

Friedlander, B. Z. A psychologist's second thoughts on concepts, curiosity, and discovery in teaching and learning. *Harvard Educational Review*, 1965, *35* (Winter) 18–37.

Gardner, J. W. *Excellence: Can we be equal and excellent too?* New York: Harper & Row, 1961.

————. *Self-renewal*. New York: Harper & Row, 1964.

Gentile, A. M. A working model of skill acquisition with application to teaching. *Quest*, 1972, Monograph *17*, 3–23.

Gezi, K., & Hadley, F. Strategies for developing critical thinking. *Journal of Nursing Education*, 1970, *9*(2), 9–13.

Hadeka, M. A., & Emerson, F. G. Alternative community placements for students: School—A good place to learn. *Nursing and Health Care*, 1982, *3*(4), 192–195.

Hagen, E. Effective use of clinical experience. Transcript of Lecture given to Nursing Education Club, Teachers College, Columbia University, November 15, 1967.

Hatrock, B. Multiple student assignments. *Nursing Outlook*, 1969, *17*(11), 40–42.

Hawkins, J. W. *Clinical experiences in collegiate nursing education*. New York: Springer Publishing, 1981.

Heidgerken, L. E. *Teaching and learning in schools of nursing*. Philadelphia: J. B. Lippincott Company, 1965.

————. This I believe . . . about a philosophy of education. *Nursing Outlook*, 1969, *17*(4), 42–43.

Highet, G. *The art of teaching*. New York: Random House, 1950.

Infante, M. S. Creating and planning clinical laboratory experiences to meet course, level, and program objectives. In *Utilization of the clinical laboratory in baccalaureate nursing programs*. New York: National League for Nursing, 1978.

Joyce, B. *The teacher and his staff: Man, media, and machines*. Washington, D.C.: National Education Association of the United States, 1967.

Keen, M. F., & Dear, M. R. Mastery of role transition: Clinical teaching strategies. *Journal of Nursing Education*, 1983, *22*(5), 183–186.

Kerlinger, F. N. *Foundations of behavioral research*. New York: Holt, Rinehart & Winston, Inc., 1973.

Kluckhohn, F., & Strodtbeck, F. *Variations in value orientations*. New York: Row Peterson and Company, 1961.

Kohn, S. D. Paolo Soleri thinks very big. *New York Times Magazine*, July 26, 1970, Section 6.

Lefkowitz, A., & Hart, A. M. Selection of laboratory facilities for collegiate nursing education. *Nursing Forum*, 1965, *4*(1), 94–102.

Leonard, B. J., & Redland, A. R. *Process in clinical nursing*. Englewood Cliffs, New Jersey: Prentice Hall, 1981.

Lindsey, M., et al. *Inquiry into teaching behavior of supervisors in teacher education laboratories*. New York: Teachers College Press, Columbia University, 1969.

Mauksch, I. G. Nurse–physician collaboration: A changing relationship. *The Journal of Nursing Administration*, 1981, *11*(6), 35–38.

McClelland, D. C. Toward a theory of motive acquisition. *American Psychologist*, 1965, *20* (April), 321–333.

McKeachie, W. J. *Teaching tips: A guide for beginning teachers*. Lexington, Massachusetts: D. C. Heath and Co., 1978.

Melera, C. B. Clinical instruction in nursing: A national survey. *Journal of Nursing Education*, 1981, *20*(8), 32–40.

Mullins, A. First clinical assignments. *Nursing Outlook*, 1965, *13* (2), 47–50.

Nishio, K. Creative problem solving: A teaching innovation. *Nursing Forum*, 1967, *6*(4), 432–441.

Olson, E. M. Baccalaureate students' perceptions of factors assisting knowledge application in the clinical laboratory. *Journal of Nursing Education*, 1983, *22*(1), 18–21.

O'Shea, H. S. Clinical instruction: Effective and ineffective teacher behaviors. *Nursing Outlook*, 1979, *27*(6), 411–415.

Petzel, R. A., Harris, I. B., & Masler, D. S. The empirical validation of clinical teaching strategies. *Evaluation and the Health Professions*, 1982, *5*(4), 499–508.

Quint, J. C. The hidden hazards in patient assignments. *Nursing Outlook*, 1965, *13*(11), 50–54.

Reilly, D. E. (Ed.). *Teaching and evaluating the affective domain in nursing programs*. New Jersey: Charles B. Slack, Inc., 1978.

———. *Behavioral objectives—Evaluation in nursing*. New York: Appleton-Century-Crofts, 1980.

Roberts, K. K., & Thurston, H. I. Teaching methodologies: Knowledge acquisition and retention. *Journal of Nursing Education*, 1984, *23*(1), 21–26.

Rogers, C. *Freedom to learn*. Columbus, Ohio: Charles E. Merrill Publishing Company, 1969.

Russell, C. H. *Liberal education and nursing*. New York: Teachers College Press, Columbia University, 1959.

Ryle, G. *The concept of mind.* London: Hutchinson House, 1949.

Saterin, J. L. Baccalaureate preparation for action—Practice nursing. *Nurse Educator,* 1978, *3*(3), 12–14.

Scheffler, I. *Conditions of knowledge.* Chicago: Scott, Foresman Company, 1965.

————. *The language of education.* Springfield, Illinois: Charles C. Thomas, 1960.

————. Philosophical models of teaching. *Harvard Educational Review,* 1965, *35* (Spring), 131–143.

Schofield, A. M., & Finnila, M. C. L. A place to explore. *Journal of Nursing Education,* 1967, *6*(3), 3–9.

Schroeder, D. M., Cantor, M. M., & Kurth, S. W. Learning needs of the new graduate entering hospital nursing. *Nurse Educator,* 1981, *6*(6), 10–17.

Schulman, J. L., Foley, J. M., & Voorsanger, E. L. Observation of a hospitalized child as a teaching technique in student nurse education. *Journal of Nursing Education,* 1966, *5* (4), 7–12, 20–21.

Schumann, D. M. An improved method of making clinical assignments. *Nursing Outlook,* 1967, *15*(4), 52–55.

Schweer, J. E., & Gelibie, K. M. *Creative teaching in clinical nursing.* St. Louis: C. V. Mosby, Co., 1976.

Silva, D., & Christy, T. A process of instruction. *Nursing Forum,* 1967, *6*(4), 419.

Singer, R. N. To err or not to err: A question for the instruction of psychomotor skills. *Review of Educational Research,* 1977, *47*(3), 479–498.

Smoyak , S. A. Teaching as coaching. *Nursing Outlook,* 1978, *26* (6), 361–363.

Taba, H. Learning by discovery. *The Elementary School Journal,* 1963, *63*(6), 308–316.

Wang, A. M., & Blumberg, P. A study on interaction techniques of nursing faculty in the clinical area. *Journal of Nursing Education,* 1983, *22*(4), 144–151.

Zanecchia, M. D. *A study of the relationships of nursing faculty attributes, faculty productivity, nursing student attributes and selected student outcomes.* Unpublished doctoral dissertation, Storrs, The University of Connecticut, 1981.

CHAPTER 4

The Process for Developing Clinical Activities

Throughout the discussion of the essential elements, reference was made to the fact that the clinical laboratory in nursing education should be used selectively to effectively accomplish the goals set for students in such a setting. The clinical laboratory then, it was established, is a culminating experience to be reserved until the latter portion of a unit of study. To proceed to the clinical laboratory, students should have demonstrated a degree of competence in the knowledge and skills demanded to be able to safely and effectively perform the expected practice with clients. This philosophical approach to teaching and learning in nursing education implies a sequence of learning activities that warrant closer examination, because the use of the clinical laboratory being proposed in this book can be accomplished only if the prerequisite set of learning activities is used by the teacher. The college laboratory that was alluded to so often in Chapter 3 is a very important part of that entire sequence of activities. So, the college laboratory and the basis for its use will be explored in some detail. Finally, the progression to the clinical laboratory with appropriate selection of clinical activities and settings is illustrated.

Use of the Conceptual Framework to Encompass and Guide Clinical Activities

Nursing education and nursing practice are moving quite successfully in the direction of using a conceptual base for action. During the past decade many studies have been taken to structure a conceptual framework that guides curricular development, modes of practice, and nursing research studies that contribute to advances in the field. A number of models [1,2,3,4] that are gaining an appreciation of and approval of educators, practitioners, and researchers have emerged; a growing sophistication in their use is evident and is leading to excitement, challenge, and accomplishment in the field. Perhaps the most exciting aspects of this phenomena are two: (1) support for the premise that a systematic use of theory leads to improved quality of practice, and (2) the professionalization of nursing is stengthened by the use of a nursing model as opposed to a medical model for practice.

In nursing education, the impressive use of conceptual models has been evident in the organization and reorganization of curricula. Emphasis on the learner and the client are striking. There has evolved a system for developing strong, theoretically based curricula that has the greatest potential for producing the type of graduates intended by nursing education, and so sorely needed by nursing service.

Interestingly enough, the conceptual framework, even where so well articulated by some faculties, has been implemented to a limited extent in the laboratory activities of the curricular plan. That is, the conceptual framework has been more fully developed in some parts of the curriculum and less fully developed in other parts. Figure 4.1 depicts the major portions of a curriculum in relation to the conceptual framework. The conceptual framework is perceived as an umbrella that permeates all aspects of the curriculum with its complementary theories, direction for practice activities, and the language to describe such activities. From the statement of philosophy of a school or department through the plan for course content, the conceptual framework is usually quite evident. Yet, in many instances, the implications and use of the framework fall short of the teaching strategies and learning activities. In laboratory settings, the framework may not be recognizable.

In the approach to the clinical laboratory being proposed, the consistent use of the conceptual framework is important. The language and the concepts should permeate all steps in the teaching/learning process. For example, if crisis theory[5] is used as a framework, the concepts of precrisis, crisis, and postcrisis, developmental and situational hazardous events, perceptions of the event, and growth will be most evident in the statement of philosophy, program objectives, course objectives, and all course content. The teaching strategies and learning activities in class, college laboratory, and clinical laboratory will center on student activities in relation to all three stages of crisis, in developmental as well as situational hazardous events, and in activities leading clients to growth. Clients perceptions of the event will be assessed as a challenge, threat, or loss, and plans for care and nursing interventions determined accordingly. Crisis theory would determine the

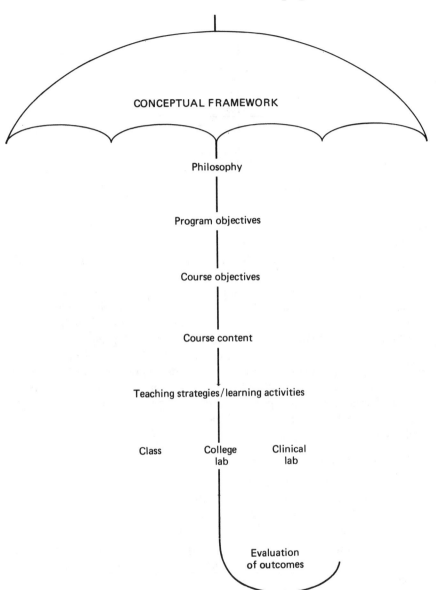

Figure 4.1 Component parts of curricular plan.

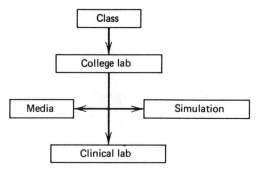

Figure 4.2 Sequence of learning activities.

age of clients that students would interact with and the settings for practice would vary accordingly. The progression of learning would follow the dictates of the theory. Theory would guide learning and learning would guide practice.

The discussion that follows assumes the use of a selected conceptual framework and sets forth a planned progression of teaching/learning activities that goes from class and class-related activities to college laboratory, and then to clinical laboratory. Figure 4.2 depicts this progression.

This sequence of learning is also consistent with the views of a philosopher of education on professional education. Phenix,[6] is perhaps best known for his categorization of learnings in the liberal arts or general education. However, he has articulated an approach to designing and organizing learnings in any professional program of study that is most meaningful to nursing. A professional curriculum, he proposes, consists of four essential components:

1. Experiences to prepare a person.
2. Sciences relevant to the profession.
3. A recasting of materials of relevant nursing science in terms of the characteristic problems of the profession. Include the function and activities of the profession, as well as the history and philosophy of that profession.
4. A consumatory study that is a practicum or case study. That which is the *craft of the profession,* or in this instance, the *craft of nursing.* Consists of:
   a. a study of the typical decisions made in the profession through case study or simulation.
   b. an actual period of practice in clinical settings.

The following discussion assumes accomplishment of the first two components and relates to the series of activities in the latter two components of the nursing curriculum—the study of the nursing major.

Classroom Activities

Classroom activities are meant to include those initial explorations of cognitive and affective learnings that occur in the classroom in the form of lectures, discussions, seminars, debates, and the like. Other related activities such as readings, written papers, and oral presentations contribute to the knowledge, understanding, and beginning transfer by students to theoretical situations. Student learning activities, coupled with appropriate teaching strategies used by the faculty member, lead the student to a readiness to acquire the attendant psychomotor skills in the area of study.

The sequence of learning implied is according to Bloom's Taxonomy of Educational Objectives for the Cognitive Domain.[7] Bloom suggests that cognitive learnings proceed as follows:

1. Knowledge
2. Understanding or comprehension
3. Application
4. Integration
5. Synthesis
6. Evaluation

In the affective domain[8] the classification scheme is as follows:

1. Receiving (attending)
2. Responding
3. Valuing
4. Organization
5. Characterization by a value or value complex

Dependent on the level of the learner in a given course in a given program of study, classroom activities support student accomplishments to an appropriate level in the cognitive and affective domains. Because nursing is heavily invested in the practice of psychomotor skills, the next step in the learning process occurs in the college laboratory.

Use of the College Laboratory

While the word *laboratory* in nursing education is often used synonymously with clinical laboratory, the college laboratory is a setting replete with its own teaching–learning strategies and that is growing in importance as an essential facet of the *nursing laboratory*. In this discussion, *college laboratory* is the term used to designate a place for students to practice skills on the college or university campus. However, some other terms in popular use that are synonymous with college laboratory are instructional laboratory, learning laboratory, and skills laboratory. Whatever the label, the exploration of the use of this portion of the nursing laboratory is intended to be the same.

The college laboratory is intended to precede the use of the clinical laboratory for each clinical laboratory objective, so that the subsequent use of the clinical laboratory assures a knowledgeable, skillful learner in each situation. Each skill objective, then, presupposes acquisition of tested knowledge, demonstration of skill in the college laboratory, and readiness for transfer of learning to the real situation. Both student and teacher must determine the level of accomplishment in the college laboratory and readiness to move to practice in the clinical laboratory.

The college laboratory needs to become an established part of the sequence of teaching–learning activities and take an important place in skill and attitude development. To do so, optimal use of the time, space, and equipment is needed. In relation to time, students should be free to practice skills when they are motivated to do so and when their personal and professional schedules permit. Hence, the suggestion is that the college laboratory be open to students during a wide range of hours, both during the week and on weekends. Also, laboratory personnel in the form of graduate assistants or baccalaureate prepared nurses in the community should be available to staff the laboratory, to serve as resource persons to the students, and to facilitate a retrieval system. Students need to have competent nurses available to guide their activities, answer questions, provide feedback to their performance, and set up the simulations needed for each set of activities. Such nurses would not teach, but would serve as valuable resources to students whenever the laboratory is open. If a lack of knowledge is determined to be the problem of a student, then the student is referred back to the faculty member for further teaching and learning before proceeding with skill acquisition. For example, if a student is learning to manipulate and assemble a syringe and medication in preparing for practicing the administration of a parenteral medication, but that student continually contaminates sterile equipment, then further study of principles of maintaining asepsis would be recommended.

Faculty members, however, need to be available in the college laboratory on much the same basis as they are available during office hours. Each faculty member makes known to the group of students, the selected hours during the week, such as, from 10 to 12 a.m. on Fridays, when he or she will be available in the laboratory to reinforce teaching, respond to questions, raise additional questions, and determine the readiness of students to move into the clinical laboratory. The faculty member's time as well as the student's time is divided between both laboratories.

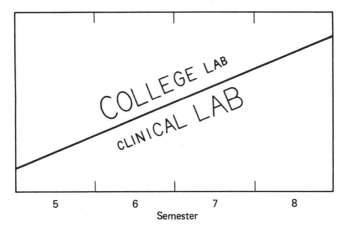

Figure 4.3 Distribution of laboratory time.

Each nursing course designates the actual number or the minimal number of laboratory hours to be devoted by each student to the practice of the psychomotor and intellectual skills of the nursing process. The total number of hours encompasses both college and clinical laboratory hours. Usually, in a given curriculum, the college laboratory and clinical laboratory hours are proportionately determined and reversed from the beginning of the program to the last semester or term. That is, the college laboratory hours typically occupy the greater proportion of time in the beginning nursing courses, and decrease in succeeding semesters until the clinical laboratory hours increase to 100 percent or nearly so in the last semester of study. Figures 4.3 and 4.4 depict two different patterns of distribution of laboratory time. The appropriate pattern should be decided on by the total faculty group teaching in a particular program.

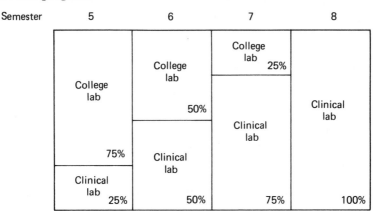

Figure 4.4 Distribution of laboratory time.

College laboratories should be designed to contain space and equipment for the viewing of media and for simulation activities. In both parts of the college laboratory, whether they are separate rooms or integrated into one setting, attention must be given to the sequence of acquiring psychomotor skills. Learning activities and evaluation techniques in this laboratory, as well as in clinical laboratory, would be designed and offered in an organized fashion. Dave's Taxonomy of Psychomotor Behaviors[9] serves as a guide.

1. Imitation

   Student follows the example or performance of another performing a skill.

2. Manipulation

   Student handles relevant equipment and assembles and tests its use.

3. Precision

   Student demonstrates performance of the skill, makes fewer errors, and aspires to accuracy.

4. Articulation

   Student coordinates a series of acts and performs the skill smoothly.

5. Naturalization

   Student achieves competency or even proficiency in performing a skill and/or a related set of skills. The particular skill performance becomes secondary to the client outcome to be achieved.

Media Laboratory.   The media portion of the college laboratory provides the environment and the equipment for the student to listen to and view the application of concepts explored in class and through readings. Either commercially or faculty produced tapes and videos portray experts involved in a skill performance to which the student aspires. Through sight and sound the learner gains a vision of what a particular performance is about, both as a whole and in its component parts. The level of imitation is possible after this set of activities.

The media laboratory is a pleasant, unhurried environment that is conducive to thinking and planning. Well-produced software provide excellent examples of role models performing a skill, such as examination of the eye. Or, audio tape of respiratory sounds and heart sounds allow the student to attune himself to normal and abnormal findings. Individual viewing and listening has distinct advantages for the student who, proceeding at his or her own pace, will review materials until there is clarity and readiness to move on. Group viewing and listening, however, also have advantages such as providing opportunity for constructive criticism, raising questions, and comparing observations.

Evidence is beginning to mount in favor of the use of mediated instruction in nursing programs. One research study[10] reports that in a quasi-experimental design one group of baccalaureate students were taught according to teacher-based instruction involving teacher demonstrations while a second group had media-based instruction. Both groups were learning physical assessment skills. No significant differences were found between media-based and teacher-based groups on measures of cognitive, affective, and psychomotor learning. The findings support the use of media-based instruction as equally effective as teacher-based methods, with significant savings in teacher time.

Simulation Laboratory.   The simulation portion of the laboratory allows for students to practice the skills themselves. In many instances, students proceed from the viewing and listening of the media laboratory to the manipulation activities of the simulation laboratory. The simulation laboratory demands the application of the intellectual and psychomotor skills of the nursing process. Simulation can be portrayed through models specifically designed and equipped for health related procedures, such as Resussci-Anne, to live staged clients. This latter type of simulation has proven to be highly useful in some areas of medical education, it seems to have much untapped potential for nursing education. Chapter 5 presents a detailed discussion of simulation.

Computers are another item that are gradually making their way into educational laboratories. For student learning, there are endless uses for computers. Training guides, instructions, opportunity for repetition and review, and self-correction, provide an optimal means of self-paced learning. Also, a terminal connection between the simulation laboratory and a clinical facility would provide updated client data for the selection of clinical activities for faculty and students. Such computer capabilities would save endless hours of commuting to clinical settings to select desirable clinical activities for students.

In the simulation laboratory, the teacher is responsible for its design and the structure of the activities to occur there. It should not be left to happenstance or the traditional design and use of the former "nursing arts" laboratories. Instead the atmosphere, layout, and plan for the activities should be planned according to principles of skill acquisition. Gentile's [11,12] work on the stages of skill acquisition provides an appropriate guide for nurse educators. In stage I, initial skill acquisition, the teacher clarifies the goal and the nature of the outcome to be produced. The student gets the idea of the movement. A set of objectives plus activities in the media laboratory assist the student to this point. The teacher is expected to fulfill three important tasks:

1. Create a specific environmental problem.
2. Establish an adequate motivational level.
3. Structure a microcosm of the total situation.

But, according to Gentile, the teacher must leave the performance of the task to the student.

A nonthreatening environment, accepting of error in trial attempts, should be fostered. Teacher comments should be delayed for a brief time so that the student can process and encode the information he obtained during and after the trial attempts.

In stage II, fixation and diversification, the teacher structures the conditions of practice and provides feedback for decision making in the future. The simulation laboratory provides ideal opportunity for stage II as well as the clinical laboratory that follows. In closed skills that are relatively easy, for example, measuring a blood pressure or making a bed, the teacher provides the same conditions as will prevail under test conditions. In open skills that are more complex, for example, changing a dressing on a draining, infected wound, the teacher varies systematically the regulatory conditions so that the student will acquire a repertoire of motor patterns as opposed to one prescribed way of behaving.

The place for student error in the learning of psychomotor skills is an intriguing concept for nurse educators. Singer[13] presents a review of the literature supporting the pros and cons of making errors. However, one conclusion is that if the purpose of the learning situation is to lead to the application of what has been learned for transfer to other related skills and situations, it would seem that some form of discovery, problem solving, or trial-and-error strategy should be employed.

In short, the college laboratory provides a wide range of opportunities for teachers of nursing to teach and for students to learn apart from the static, rigors, and demands of the clinical settings. It is a change to practice apart from pressure before performing in a real situation. The suggestion is not to use the college laboratory in lieu of clinical laboratory time; instead, the suggestion that an appropriate balance be struck between the two and that each be used for a specified purpose—allow one to lead to and complement the other.

The following exercise is presented to illustrate the difference in and the progression from the students' activities in the college laboratory and in the clinical laboratory.

Statement of Objectives

Carries out selective interventions to relieve various types of respiratory distress.

College Laboratory Activities

Listen to tapes on normal/abnormal lung sounds.

Observes films on assessment of lungs and upper respiratory passages.

Reviews films depicting airway obstruction of various types and stages.

Identifies various types of respiratory distress.

Performs assessments of respiratory tract on peers.

Performs assessment of respiratory tract on simulated client (that is, simulated for emphysema).

Formulates nursing diagnoses.

Tests a selected nursing intervention.

Records findings accurately.

Manipulates various devices used to relieve respiratory distress, that is, aerosol sprays, respirators.

Clinical Laboratory Activities

Conducts respiratory assessments on selected clients.

Assesses three clients with chronic obstructive lung disease in varying stages and at differing ages.

Assesses three clients experiencing acute respiratory distress ranging in age from a child to an older adult.

Arrives at nursing diagnoses.

Records findings in a format that is in accordance with the conceptual framework in use.

Determines nursing interventions in each situation.

Renders interventions wherever possible.

Compares and contrasts findings and client outcomes at clinical conference.

Such a use of college and clinical laboratory suggests a particular use of clinical conferences. Actually, preclinical conferences with a group of students tends to become unnecessary. Individual preclinical conference to plan clinical activities for a week or two at a time becomes more useful. Students and faculty discuss what has been accomplished in relation to stated objectives, what remains to be accomplished, and what resources might be used to accomplish their goals. At stated intervals, perhaps every two weeks, a postclinical conference serves the purpose of students sharing experiences and comparing impressions. Peer input into future planning can also be encouraged.

These postclinical conferences need to be of sufficient length to provide time for thoughtful reporting and discussion. A typical length might be two hours. Also, the faculty member should lead the conference in such a manner as to probe the meaning of what was learned and tease the imagination of the students for what might be learned. Attention might be given to:

1. Comparing and contrasting findings and outcomes among clients (include age, setting, and level of wellness).
2. Proposing alternate nursing interventions.
3. Applying criteria to determine effectiveness and efficiency of outcomes.
4. Probing attitudinal dimensions.
5. Soliciting suggestions for future learnings and clinical activities.

Student participation should be heightened; teacher activities amount to subtle suggestion and leadership. Postclinical conferences should extend and enhance classroom learnings and college laboratory activities through the sharing of actual client encounters placed within a purposeful context.

Summary

The use of the college laboratory as suggested in this chapter serves as a bridge between classroom learnings and clinical activities. The purposes of such a design for college laboratory are to:

Increase the effectiveness and efficiency of time spent by nursing students with clients.

Produce a more knowledgeable and skillful student for the clinical laboratory.

Provide a sensible, sequential progression from class to clinical laboratory.

Make for better use of the faculty member's time.

Provide a more accurate picture of the rate of progression of students.

Reduce student anxiety in the initial learning of psychomotor skills by structuring an environment free from static.

Notes

1. Riehl, J. P., & Roy, C. *Conceptual models for nursing practice.* New York: Appleton-Century-Crofts, 1980.
2. Orem, D. E. *Nursing: Concepts of practice.* New York: McGraw-Hill, 1980.
3. Travelbee, J. *Interpersonal aspects of nursing.* Philadelphia: F. A. Davis Company, 1971.

4. Neuman, B. M., & Young, R. J. A model for teaching total person approach to patient problems. *Nursing Research,* 1972, *21,* (3) 264–269.

5. Infante, M. S. (Ed.). *Crisis theory: A framework for nursing practice.* Reston, Virginia: Reston Publishing Company, 1982.

6. Phenix, P. H. *Realms of meaning.* New York: McGraw-Hill Book Company, 1964.

7. Bloom, B. S. (Ed.). *Taxonomy of educational objectives. Cognitive domain.* New York: David McKay Company, Inc., 1956.

8. Krathwohl, D. R., Bloom, B. S., & Masia, B. B. *Taxonomy of educational objectives. Affective domain.* New York: David McKay Company, Inc., 1964.

9. Dave, R. H. Psychomotor levels. In *Developing and writing behavioral objectives.* Tucson, Arizona: Educational Innovators Press, 1970, p. 33.

10. Utz, S. W., Hayward, M. B., Zachman, R., & Utz, R. A comparison of teacher-based and media-based instruction in teaching physical assessment skills to undergraduate nursing students. Medical College of Ohio (Unpublished study).

11. Gentile, A. M. A working model of skill acquisition with application to teaching. *Quest,* 1972, Monograph 17.

12. ———. Structure of motor tasks in Mouvement Actes du 7th symposium in apprentissage psycho moteur et psychologie du sport, October 1975, 11–28.

13. Singer, R. N. To err or not to err: A question for the instruction of psychomotor skills. *Review of Educational Reserach,* 1977, *47,* (3), 479–498.

Bibliography

Bitzer, M. Clinical nursing instruction via PLATO simulated laboratory. *Nursing Research,* 1966, *15* (2), 144–150.

Burrell, S. L. O. *The effectiveness of self-assessment guides as a method of teaching critical care nursing to professional nursing students.* Athens, Georgia: unpublished doctoral dissertation, University of Georgia, 1978.

Dowling, G. R. *A study of teaching in pre- and postconferences of clinical nursing courses.* Unpublished doctoral dissertation, Teachers College, Columbia University, 1970.

Farrell, J. J. Media in the nursing curriculum. *Nurse Educator,* 1981, *6,* (4), 15–19.

Fleming, M. Characteristics of effective instructional presentation: What we know and what we need to know. *Educational Technology,* 19, *21* (7), 33–38.

Gaevert, H. Striking a balance between content and method in nursing education. *Nursing Forum,* 1978, *17* (3), 245–257.

Gagné, R. *The condition of learning.* New York: Holt, Rinehart, & Winston, Inc., 1970.

Griffin, G. J. *Clinical nursing instruction by television.* New York: Bureau of Publications, Teachers College, Columbia University, 1965.

Guzzetta, C. E. Relationship between stress and learning. *Advances in Nursing Science,* 1979, *1* (4), 35–48.

Hill, E. J. M. *A study of the verbal interaction between master teachers and students during clinical nursing conference.* Unpublished doctoral dissertation, Teachers College, Columbia University, 1967.

Huckabay, L. *Conditions of learning and instruction in nursing.* St. Louis: C. V. Mosby Co., 1980.

Kissinger, J. F., & Munjas, B. A. Nursing process, student attributes, and teaching methodologies. *Nursing Research,* 1981, *30* (4), 242–246.

Knowles, M. S. *The adult learner: A neglected species.* Houston: Gulf Publishing Co., 1973.

––––––. *The modern practice of adult education: Androgogy vs. pedagogy.* New York: Associated Press, 1975.

Machlup, F. Poor learning from good teachers. *Academe,* 1979, *65* (6), 376–380.

Matheney, R. V. Pre- and postconferences for students. *American Journal of Nursing,* 1969, *69* (2), 286–289.

McLuhan, M. *Understanding media: The extension of man.* New York: McGraw-Hill Book Company, Inc., 1964.

McPhetridge, L. Three methods of conducting a nursing skills lab. *Nursing Research,* 1968, *17* (5), 462–463.

Mirin, S. K. *Teaching tomorrow's nurse: A nurse educator reader.* Wakefield, Massachusetts: Nursing Resources, Inc., 1980.

Munro, M. F. *The use of written simulations to measure problem-solving skills of nursing students.* Unpublished doctoral dissertation, The University of Michigan, 1979.

Murray, L. M. A comparison of lecture–discussion and self-study methods in nursing education. *Journal of Nursing Education,* 1982, *21* (9), 17–23.

Paduano, M. A. Bringing about learning in the college laboratory. *Journal of Nursing Education,* 1978. *17* (6), 30–33.

Peterson, P. L., & Walberg, H. J. (Eds.). *Research on teaching: Concepts, findings, and implications.* Berkeley, California: McCutchan Publishers, 1979.

Plummer, E. M. The clinical conference discussion leader. *Nursing Forum,* 1974, *13* (1), 94–104.

Sullivan, K. From learning modules to clinical practice. *Nursing Outlook,* 1977, *25* (5), 319–321.

Utz, S. W., Hayward, M. B., Zachman, R., & Utz, R. A comparison of teacher-based and media-based instruction in teaching physical assessment skills to undergraduate nursing students. Toledo, Ohio, Medical College of Ohio (Unpublished study).

Weaver, R. L. Effective lecturing techniques: Alternatives to classroom boredom. *Teacher Educator*, 1980, 5 (1), 2–8.

Wofl, Z. R. et al. How useful is the preclinical conference? *Nursing Outlook*, 1979, 27 (7), 455–457.

CHAPTER 5

Simulation as a Strategy for Teaching in the College Laboratory

Definition of and Use of Simulation

In the broadest sense, simulation is a replication of the essential aspects of reality so that the reality can be better understood, controlled, and practiced. A simulation is used for a specific purpose or goal. For example, the goal may be to acquire knowledge, gain a skill, or change attitudes. Simulation is characterized by accuracy and by comprehensiveness in that it includes a range of dimensions. The simulation itself can take many forms depending on the learning goal. The first recorded educational use of simulation came out of Germany in 1789. It took the form of a complex war game and provided a model for subsequent military simulated exercises. Such exercises continue to be a standard and essential component of military training. Simulation continues to allow officers and trainees a chance to gain experience in strategy and tactics without loss of life.

In the 1930s role playing as another variety of simulation was introduced into educational settings. Here the goal was to improve interactions between

---

This chapter was contributed by Wendy J. Fibison, R.N., B.S., M.H.Sc., C.R.N., P.N.P., an Instructor of Nursing at the University of Connecticut and doctoral candidate at the University of Pennsylvania, Genetics Graduate Group.

people. One of the early mechanical simulations was the dummy aircraft cockpit that simulated flight conditions. Space technology has elaborated on the theme. The 1950s saw the business world develop yet another variation, that of high finance games. Commercial managers could practice decision making without risking bankruptcy. Recent advances in computer technology have resulted in sophisticated computerized simulations.[1]

As a teaching strategy simulation fosters student involvement and increases interest and motivation. The focus becomes the learning instead of pleasing the instrument, object, or recipient. The student can experience the problem or situation from a variety of perspectives and orientations. A simulation allows the student to analyze the elements of a problem and their relationships to one another. Relationships between theory and action or behavior can be made free from the pressure and demands of a real setting. Also, providing a common experience, participants can learn from one another. Simulations require student decision making and foster self-awareness, as well as self-correction.

Simulation as a teaching strategy has been used in nursing education for years. "Mrs. Chase" could almost be categorized as a rite of passage for nursing students. In the literature simulation is often used synonymously with game, but it is necessary to distinguish between them. Simulation has already been defined; however, a game is an activity performed by cooperating or competing decision makers seeking to achieve a goal within a set of rules. There is a predetermined end point. The learning objective can be cognitive, or it can focus on the application of knowledge. Games can also be used for evaluative purposes. As with simulations, games require active participation, foster interaction and peer learning, and allow students to test knowledge in a nonthreatening, nongraded situation.

The teaching strategy simulation game provides elements from both. McKenzie[2] defines a simulation game as an "activity of decision makers who are seeking to gain objectives, under the constraint of rules, in a make-believe world." Aspects of the real world are mimicked in a structured game format with rules, goals, activities, resources, limitations, and rewards. Simulations, games, and simulation games offer nursing education effective techniques for challenging students. Such techniques may take different forms.

Case analysis is one form of simulation that has been used widely and can be an effective strategy for developing decision-making skills. For example, Erickson and Borgmeyer[3] describe the use of simulated nursing administration situations.

> At 3:30 p.m., Ms. A., the director of nursing, had just returned to her office at the hospital from the local nurse facilitator monthly conference and luncheon. A note on the door stated that Ms. D., the administrator, would

like to see her immediately on return. After checking other relevant messages, Ms. A. went to the administrator's office.

The secretary motioned her to go directly in as Ms. D. was waiting. "Mrs. A., are you aware of the condition of Ms. T. when she reported for duty today?" Confessing ignorance, Ms. A. explained that she had just returned from a conference outside the hospital and was not aware of any problem. "Well, you are going to have to do something as it is obvious that Ms. T. is inebriated. According to policy, she should be automatically terminated. Please take care of it and report back."

Additional background data about the hospital and individuals is provided. Students apply the Bailey/Claus[4] decision-making model and, through retrospective examination of this actual problem, analyze goals and constraints, generate alternatives and approaches, and define decision criteria. Students choose and implement a course of action and evaluate the results. The authors conclude that the reality orientation to simulated decision making provides an effective teaching–learning strategy in nursing service administration education.

Case analysis as a form of simulation can also be in the form of a patient assessment and management problem. The focus of learning becomes discriminating between necessary and unnecessary information, interpreting data, planning interventions, and monitoring the results.

Corbett and Beveridge[5] describe use of the clinical case simulation in conjunction with the clinical laboratory experience. Before their clinical day begins, students "take care of" a simulated case. The case is similar to the actual patients the students will be caring for, and provides a focus for postconference. Because all students have cared for the same patient, participation tends to be active. Being a risk-free situation, students openly discuss their mistakes and critique each other's approach. Additionally, case simulations can also be used in the classroom to organize discussion of nursing theory. Barrows and Tamblyn[6] developed a unique variation of the case simulation. It is called P_4, Portable Patient Problem Pack, and is a method of simulating a patient's problem in a card deck format.[6] It consists of a deck of 3″ by 5″ cards in a variety of colors. Each color designates the type of action that can be taken with the patient: white for interview questions; blue for items on physical examination; orange for investigations, laboratory tests, and diagnostic procedures; green for consultants; pink for nursing and medical interventions; yellow for situation and closure. Additional cards with photographs can be added. On the front of each card in capital letters is the specific action that the card represents. Some examples are shown in Table 5.1. Below the card title are questions that the student should ask before turning the card over to read the response. For example, if the physical examination (blue) card for lungs were chosen, the student must answer the following questions before turning the card over.

TABLE 5.1. Examples of Card Titles in the Color Categories

Type of Action	Color	Card Titles
Interview questions	White	How did your problem start and when?
		Why are you here today?
		Any precipitating or aggravating factors?
		What was done in the past about your problem?
		Respiratory system review
		Allergies?
		Past or present life stresses?
		How does your problem affect your daily life?
		Habits—sleep, exercise, drinking, smoking
		Developmental history
Physical examination	Blue	General appearance
		Vital signs
		Respiratory system
		Cardiovascular system
Investigations	Orange	Chest x-ray
		Skin testing
		Urinalysis
		Hemoglobin/hematocrit
Consultants	Green	Respirologist
		Clinical psychologist
		Pharmocologist
		Clinical nurse specialist
		Community nurse
		Spouse, parents, children, friends
Interventions	Pink	Tepid sponge
		Bronchodilators
		Vaporizer
		Force fluids
		Community nursing
		Patient education
		Modification of life style

Why did you select this card?

Could you perform this examination?

Can you interpret the possible results from this examination?

How would positive or negative findings influence your hypothesis?

Do you understand the principles or facts in human biology to evaluate any findings?

If a consultant card is chosen, the following questions must be answered.

Why select this card?

How does it relate to your hypothesis?

What information will you communicate to the consultant?

What request will you make of the consultant?

These questions are designed to help the student develop effective and efficient problem-solving skills. On the backs of the cards are responses to the action indicated: answers to interview questions, physical examination findings, results of invesitagions, and opinions of consultants.

Results of interventions are described, as the case is based on an actual patient situation. There are many more cards in each category than are actually needed for problem solving. This provides the student with a wide range of actions from which to choose, and avoids cueing the student by including only pertinent cards. The cards are situated so that all titles can be seen. The situation card is read. The following situation is from a P_4 designed for students in a nursing practitioner program.[7]

> A child is brought to your office by his mother because he has a cold and is having difficulty breathing.

The student decides what action to take first, whether it be asking a question or taking vital signs. The questions pertaining to the action are addressed and the result is read. The student continues in this matter until the problem is solved. At any time the process may be stopped so that the student can consult with peers, faculty, or the literature. The closure card is chosen when the student has completed the assessment and management. Questions on the closure card are:

What have you decided this diagnosis is?

What were your differentials?

Did you find out what the family structure is?

Does this have implications for long-term management?

What would you tell the family regarding his long-term prognosis?

Write a problem list for this case study.

Chart in problem-oriented record form.

Cards are stacked in order of choice, and at the end the student's cognitive pathway they can be reviewed. This simulation format can be used to meet several objectives: (1) to develop problem-solving skills; (2) to assist the student in identifying learning needs, (3) to foster self-directed study, and (4) to evaluate a student's ability to assess and manage a problem. A detailed description of this strategy, including methods of scoring, are presented by Barrows and Tamblyn.[6]

The *written simulation* as a teaching strategy for nursing was described in 1968 by deTornyay.[8] A patient situation is provided and after reviewing it, the student responds to a series of questions. A paper-and-pencil simulation possesses certain characteristics. It is an actual nursing situation. The exercise requires a series of sequential, interdependent decisions that represent the various steps in the nursing process. The student receives feedback after each decision. Should an action prove ineffectual or harmful, it is possible to revise the action. The problem can accommodate a variety of approaches. This teaching strategy allows the focus to be on selected problem-solving skills without the constraints imposed by the clinical setting and the needs of real patients.

In reviewing the use of the written simulation, Page[9] notes that the skills focus can be in any of the following areas: assessing priorities, eliciting data, interpreting data, efficiency, use of resources, deciding on interventions, evaluating outcomes, and ordering an action sequence. It is safe to assume that as computer technology is used more in nursing education, the written simulation is destined to become computerized. Taylor[10] reported research evaluating computer simulations for nursing education.

Role playing, another form of simulation, provides for the taking of the role of a person in real life. Or it may be that a role played in real life is experienced. Human interaction and spontaneity are key elements of this strategy. It can take a variety of forms. Perhaps the most traditional use is when a student assumes the role of the patient and acts out a specific behavior while another student acts as nurse. While they interact, the other class members observe, analyze, and then give feedback. Both the *actors* and the *audience* report significant learnings and share their new insights into the subject matter.

Role playing may be extended to a family situation. Still another variation is to have the student role play a patient with a physical limitation and attempt to accomplish activities of daily living. For example, one of the nursing students may be assigned to go through the cafeteria with a blindfold or in a wheelchair. Students can also role play certain feelings, such as anxiety or anger, while classmates attempt to identify the feeling being portrayed. The latter fosters a keener awareness of nonverbal communication. A rather unique use of role playing was described by Keller and MacCormick.[11] Graduate nursing students were learning about curriculum development. They assumed faculty and administrative roles and during a semester they designed a curriculum. This provided students an opportunity to test future roles in a safe, nonthreatening environment. All participants were impressed by how significantly personal values and beliefs affected the group task; how much the process of curriculum development must be appreciated as well as the content of it. Also, it became apparent that trust had to be developed if they were going to accomplish the task. These are lessons that are difficult to convey via the lecture mode of teaching.

Simulations also include *audiovisual resources,* such as films, tapes, and simulators. Cardiac simulators produce realistic heart sounds and representative EKGs. Records and tapes have been made of breath sounds. Both assist the student to identify the elements of the sounds produced, such as pitch, intensity, and timing. Use of these audio simulations can be used in conjunction with discussion of related anatomy and physiology. Because abnormal sounds are also part of the simulations, the student can learn to distinguish normal from abnormal. Beside teaching a basic assessment skill such as assessment of breath or heart sounds, the use of audio simulations can provide students with an appreciation for the variation in describing these sounds. In a classroom setting, all students listen to the same breath or heart sound. Each student writes a description of the sound and then these are shared. The wide variation of terms used, the different interpretations of short and prolonged, and so forth, usually surprise students. The ensuing dicussion can focus on the definition of terms and rationale for the different choices, or it can focus on handling the interpersonal situation when two listeners hear the same sound differently.

Another valuable audiovisual aid used in simulation is videotaping. Videotaping is a resource that is frequently used to teach interpersonal skills. It may be an observational experience. Students view a simulated nurse–patient interpersonal situation and then analyze elements, hypothesize outcomes, evaluate outcomes, and suggest alternative approaches. Gerrard and Buzzell[12] developed an elaborate simulated videotape to be used to give students a sense of experiencing difficult interpersonal situations. From an extensive survey of health professionals, a variety of commonly encountered interpersonal problem situations were identified. These involved health professionals, patients, and student evaluators. Actors and actresses were scripted to portray the various situations. Each situation was staged as if the student were being addressed directly. The student views the video and responds directly to the challenge. Evaluation criteria have been developed and can be used by a student observer to objectively evaluate the student's interpersonal skills. A demonstration tape, a description of the development of this simulation tool, suggestions for use, and evaluation criteria are available through Reston Publishing Company, 11480 Sunset Hills Road, Reston, VA 22090.

Games can be used for a variety of cognitive, psychomotor, or evaluative learning objections. New facts may be learned or previously learned material recalled. Facts may need to be reordered or reinterpreted. Games can be a vehicle for changing attitudes or practicing intellectual or psychomotor skills. Self, peer, or formal evaluation can be accomplished through the use of games. In a broader sense, games foster acceptance of competing interests, and hopefully, how to be a generous winner or gracious loser. Most importantly, games demonstrate how to conduct a process more effectively.

One game designed to increase student knowledge is called "Positive Pressure."[13] It measures concepts related to common respiratory disease. Cards, each listing the name of a disease, symptomatology, pathophysiology, and treatment and nursing care, are matched to form a set of four correct combinations. Correct matching is facilitated by color coding each category (for example, all symptomology cards are blue). The games ends when all the cards have been grouped in fours. Five other games are described by the authors, along with the general concept measured, the cognitive style of learning that is facilitated by the game, and student responses to use of the game in the classroom.[13]

"Pill Review" is a game that was devised for evaluative purposes.[14] It tests knowledge about commonly used psychotropic drugs. A box of labeled pills is passed around. Each student blindly selects one and must name two facts about the pill, such as chemical grouping or action. If unable to do so, another student may challenge and if he or she correctly names two items, takes the pill away from the first holder. The winner is the one with the most pills at the end of the game.

Games have a wide variety of uses in evaluation, both in the cognitive and psychomotor skill domains. Beyond uses in formal educational programs, games can be used for evaluation in inservice or continuing education programs. For example, after an inservice program on hypertension in a senior center, participants played a game. Correct answers lowered the blood pressure on a scoreboard. The winning team was the one who attained the lowest blood pressure.[15]

The *teaching strategy simulation game* draws on elements from both simulations and games. Reality is structured into a game format with rules, goals, activities, resources, constraints, and payoffs. "Humanization" by *Motive* is one example.[16] Each player takes on the identity of a patient in a mental institution. The goals are to attain a place to live and a job as quickly as possible. The obstacles on the game board are the difficulties encountered in achieving these goals. A simulation game such as this could be used to help prepare the student to deal more insightfully and emphathetically with psychiatric patients about to reenter society. "Life-Cycle: A Social-Simulation Game" was designed to improve attitudes and communication skills of service providers when they interact with the elderly.[17] It can be played by nurses, medical students, nursing home administrators, nurses' aides, chaplains, or volunteers. It combines a board game with role-playing and affords learners the chance to step prematurely into a simulated age and into situations that are common in the lives of the sick elderly. Research has shown this simulation game to be effective in improving attitudes toward the elderly.[18] An instruction booklet and videotape, or slide/tape demonstration, which are part of the teaching package, describe the rules of the game and the gaming process in detail. The rules are also summarized and published in the supplement 1977 issue of *Health Education Monographs*.

A few selected examples of simulations, games, and simulation games that are used in nursing education are provided by way of illustration of the use of these teaching strategies. There are both advantages and disadvantages to using such strategies.

Advantages and Disadvantages of the Simulation Technique

Simulation techniques can be used to meet a variety of objectives: cognitive, attitudinal, or psychomotor. They may be used for both teaching, and evaluation purposes. Students are provided an opportunity to test knowledge in a safe and controlled environment. Student participation is active and these strategies tend to increase interest, involvement, and motivation. Interaction between participants fosters peer learning. Students are required to make decisions and then receive immediate feedback on their actions. The focus on decision making can proceed without the distraction of having to handle all the competing needs encountered in the clinical laboratory setting. Further, it is well known that it is difficult for a teacher to assess certain skills in the clinical laboratory due to faculty–student ratios, type of clients available, and the needs and constraints of the situation, time, and space. Simulations can be used to teach and evaluate a variety of these skills. Simulations allow students to view and experience a problem from a variety of perspectives. And most importantly, simulations place the emphasis on individual learning.

But simulation as a teaching strategy is not without disadvantages. Simulations and games take time to develop and require testing. If they are not well designed or explained, they may not be valid, that is, teach what they were intended to teach. A game may be too complicated and require extensive explanation, or it may take too long to play. In certain situations, students may disclose more about themselves than they are comfortable with. Or the experience may be so much *fun* that faculty and students become anxious about the quality of learning that has occurred. Use of simulations in the classroom and in the college laboratory changes the role of the faculty member from lecturer to that of facilitator. Although highly desirable, formal preparation for this role is needed. Change to such a style of teaching can be difficult for some.

As with any teaching strategy, careful preparation must precede its use. The learning objective needs to be carefully defined. Then begins the work of choosing the appropriate strategy. What does the strategy teach? How well does it teach in comparison to other methods? How effective is the learning? A variety of other factors also need to be considered: cost, space and equipment requirements, maintenance needs, preparation time required, the number of students that can participate at any time, the length of time needed to play, debriefing needs, and student acceptance. Careful consideration of all these factors will insure a choice that meets the educational objective and can readily be incorporated into the program.

New directions in nursing practice necessitate new teaching strategies. The trend is to expand the range of basic skills to include completing a health history, conducting a health assessment, and counseling. It is important to provide students with the opportunity to learn these skills before they assume client care responsibilities. One way to accomplish this is through the use of the simulated patient in the college laboratory setting. To date, most of the experience with this teaching strategy has been in medical education. It has equally great potential for application to nursing education, both graduate and undergraduate. The remainder of this chapter is designed to focus on the definition of the simulated client, uses, advantages, and disadvantages of the method, and the process of simulation in nursing education. A sample case for simulation is subsequently presented. The last section focuses on research—research that has evaluated the simulated client as a teaching strategy, and the potential for further research on the use of this strategy in nursing education.

The Simulated Client or Patient

In this section the word *patient* will be used instead of client because the literature in this area uses the term *simulated patient*. A simulated patient is a "healthy person who has been carefully trained to simulate the historical, physical, and emotional features of an actual patient with sufficient realism to prevent detection by experienced clinicians."[19] It should be noted specifically that real patient situations provide the material for simulations. The *healthy person* can be practically any age and usually simulates a real patient within the same age range. A well-trained simulated patient placed in a clinical setting would be mistaken for an actual patient by the health professional conducting the interview and physical examination. Talented and experienced simulated patients become proficient in portraying emotions and exhibiting physical signs. This concept can be extended to a family when such is the unit of study.

The Process of Simulating a Patient

Because realism without risk is a major feature of the simulated patient, this is an excellent strategy to prepare the student for actual patient care responsibilities. There are a variety of ways the simulated patient can be used to accomplish this overall goal.

Uses of the Simulated Patient.   The simulated patient (SP) can provide opportunity for the student to develop interviewing skills and physical assessment skills. Use may focus on the development of sound, effective, and efficient problem-solving skills. Experience with an SP may be used as a springboard for discussion in the classroom setting. If, during the course of education, the student has not had experience with a certain type of learning situation, for example, communication with a person facing death from advanced cancer, an SP, so scripted, can provide an important element of that experience. It can be an ideal strategy for evaluation purposes. And finally, it is a strategy that can be useful in educational and clinical research.

Because the SP has assumed the identity of a real patient with respect to historical data, presentation of self, and emotional characteristics, the SP can provide the student with an opportunity to develop or refine interviewing skills. While interviewing the SP, the student can focus on any number of the elements of interviewing. The beginning student may use the activity to practice self-introduction, and to practice formulating questions that are clear and in terms that the patient can understand. Organization of questions may be a focus for another student. A more advanced student may use the activity to improve her ability to detect nonverbal cues. Controlling the interview may be the focus, or the student may try new approaches to handling the uncooperative patient—the angry patient, the depressed patient, or the patient who does not want help. The particular focus chosen with respect to interviewing skills will depend on the learning objective for the session and the student's needs.

The structure of this learning experience will depend on faculty–student ratios, available facilities, and equipment. The instructor may interview the SP in front of a large class for the purpose of demonstrating interviewing skills. Students are responsible for observing the interview and identifying specific skills exhibited by the interviewer, such as clarifying the patient's complaint, active listening, or use of silence. Student responses may be verbal or written. In a small group setting (six to nine students), each student may be required to interview the patient for five minutes, starting where the previous student ended. The students observe the interviewing student and plan their approach. A student may detect a missed nonverbal cue, "You seem to find it difficult to sit still," and pursue its meaning. Or if a symptom was not completely explored, this may be returned to.

In other situations, the student may believe that the major problem has been missed and launch into a whole new focus of inquiry. When the observing students do not identify omissions, ineffective approaches, or any other lack of interviewing skill, the instructor can facilitate this "discovery" by asking the students appropriate questions. Another way to structure this activity in a small group is to have a student volunteer to begin the interview. The interviewer continues until becoming "stuck". At this point, the interviewer may call a "time out" and obtain helpful suggestions from the other students and the instructor on how to proceed. The same student may proceed, incorporating these ideas, or another student may volunteer to contine the interview. Regardless of which structure is used, the interview can be stopped at any point for discussion. The pause may be student or instructor initiated. The discussion may focus on "what is good," "what is not working," or "what cues the patient is giving you that tells you something is not right."

The SP has been trained to expect "time outs" and to not let the discussion alter his or her behavior. The SP has been instructed to respond only to interviewing styles and techniques, not to discussion content. This response is in keeping with the real patient's character. For example, if a student asks a sensitive question too early in the interview, the SP responds appropriately. Likewise, if a student is skillful at defusing anger, the SP becomes calmer.

At the conclusion of the interview and discussion, the SP gives feedback to each student who participated. The SP identifies how it "felt" to be that student's patient and what in the student's behavior and interviewing technique contributed to that feeling. Feedback includes positive and negative feelings. It does not include suggestions for what would have made the interview better. That is left for the student to think about. The role of the SP in providing feedback is strictly to articulate feelings and to identify what student behaviors were responsible for creating or amplifying them.

When an SP is used to teach interviewing skills, the primary role of the teacher is that of facilitator. This role is accomplished in a variety of ways. The instructor briefs and debriefs the SP. Briefing and debriefing is extremely important and is explained in detail in a later section. The instructor sets the stage by reviewing the learning objectives, describing the structure, and explaining the patient situation. Once the interviewing has begun, the instructor helps students to identify effective and less-than-effective interviewing techniques. The instructor supports the interviewing student as necessary. At the same time, the instructor assists the observing students to identify other approaches or techniques that may lead to increased effectiveness. The instructor also guides the feedback of the SP. An SP may have difficulty identifying a feeling or articulating it in a manner useful to the student. At the end of the activity, the instructor summarizes the learning and points the students to new directions of learning.

Use of the SP for teaching interviewing skills has been reported in the literature.[20-24] This experience has occurred primarily in medical schools. One such experience can be found in the Department of Obstetrics and Gynecology at the University of Edinburgh, Scotland.[25] Convinced that good interviewing skills were essential to the practice of reproductive medicine and that the SP could help students learn these skills, physician educators developed a program for undergraduate medical students. Objectives were developed in behavioral terms that students were expected to attain by the end of their rotation in reproductive medicine. Then the most common reproductive health needs of the community were identified: (1) women pregnant and planning to continue the pregnancy, (2) women who wished to terminate a pregnancy, (3) women wanting contraception, (4) women who had been unable to conceive, (5) women with menstrual disorders, (6) miscellaneous gynecologic complaints, and (7) men and women with sexual concerns. For each of these categories, competencies that would be expected to be demonstrated by the students were defined. As an example, competencies related to the problem of an unwanted pregnancy were articulated as follows:

1. Recognizes the problems of the woman with an unwanted pregnancy, her feelings and concerns about abortion or the continuation of her pregnancy, and assists her to clarify her ambivalence.
2. Advises her on the method of abortion indicated and its risk factors.
3. Advises her on the health professional support available if her pregnancy is to continue.
4. Assists her to recover from abortion and to plan any future pregnancies.

Skills in communication were identified as a priority if these competencies were to be achieved. It was also appreciated that reproductive issues are very sensitive ones, necessitating skill in handling patients who are experiencing anger, distress, grief, ambivalence. The interviewer may meet with aggression or silence and withdrawal or garrulity. The physician educators felt a responsibility to have students demonstrate competence with an SP before being involved with actual patients. They simulated a number of representative cases and used the SPs in a variety of structured formats. The SP would be interviewed in an "office" while faculty and other classmates observed through a two-way mirror. With the instructor as facilitator, a small group of students jointly interviewed an SP. In another instance, each student interviewed a different SP and then all the students gathered to compare their experiences. In evaluating this approach to education in reproductive medicine, the educators were enthusiastic about the SP as a teaching strategy. As a result, they believed that students were better equipped to meet the interpersonal challenges with real patients. Many related patient care issues that previously had been neglected in the program, arose quite naturally from the experiences with the SP. Interestingly, it also was noted that by using SPs a more representative range of patients could be presented to the students.

At Case Western Reserve University, the medical school used the SP stragegy in the unit on sexuality.[26] Students participated in the three facets of the program: (1) explicit films/small group discussions, (2) a 12-hour lecture course, and (3) a supervised videotaped interview of an SP. Pre- and posttesting showed that medical students anticipate greater discomfort and less skill in this subject area than with general medical interviewing. After the simulated patient unit, significant positive changes occurred in the students' comfort and view of their skills. It could be anticipated that these students would be less likely to avoid this area of history taking in the future now that they were more comfortable with the subject area.

Problems in communication among health professionals and patients or parents of a child with a fatal illness are well recognized. One program demonstrated that pediatric residents, with limited instruction, can be taught to give bad news to parents using effective information giving and interpersonal skills.[27] The program on "Simulated Parents" was the teaching strategy. Use of the program had three objectives:

1. To provide instruction to residents in critical information to discuss with the parents during the first interview.
2. To provide instruction and give feedback to the residents on interpersonal and communication skills that enhance their effectiveness in crises interactions with parents.
3. To evaluate the program's effectiveness in improving the resident's information giving and interpersonal skills.

The above was developed for use on the hematology/oncology rotation. The actual patient situations used for the simulations were families with a child who had been newly diagnosed with acute lymphocytic leukemia. The simulated parents were professional counselors. There were three components to the program. After a brief orientation, residents were given a lecture on the important aspects of childhood leukemia or a comprehensive handout summarizing the information. This was followed by two 90-minute sessions with the simulated parents. The first was during the first week of rotation and a second session with different simulated parents during the last week. During these sessions, the resident had 30 minutes to inform the simulated parents that their child had leukemia. The session was videotaped. After this interview, the resident completed a checklist identifying the critical information that had been imparted to the parents. Meanwhile, the simulated parents completed a checklist that identified their feeling during the session and a second checklist in which they rated the clarity of the information that the resident had imparted. Then the resident and the parents reviewed the checklists and the videotape. The simulated parents provided constructive feedback to the resident. At the end, the resident completed an evaluation form, rating the session as a learning experience. The component of the second session at the end of the rotation was essentially the same. Results of the study were as follows: residents improved in the amount of essential or critical information they imparted to the parents during the interview, clarity of the imparted information improved, the number of residents who were rated as having an overall acceptable positive level of interpersonal skills increased, and the residents rated the learning strategy as "effective" to "very effective." Another finding identified two important skill areas that needed improvement: listening to the parents and enlisting parental participation in the child's treatment program.

Other reports in the literature[28,29] describe the use of the simulated patient for teaching interviewing skills. At McMaster University self-directed learning, problem-based learning, and small group tutorials are features of the approach to medical education.[30] To accomplish the goals of the program, extensive learning resources have been developed. Use of the SP figures in prominently. Table 5.2 is a list of simulations designed specifically for teaching interviewing skills at McMaster University. Faculty, or students decide which SP will best meet the learning needs at that particular time, and they make arrangements to interview the SP that is chosen.

Another use of the SP is for the teaching of physical assessment skills. It is remarkable to note the wide range of anatomic and physiologic dysfunctions that have been synthesized. The skillful SP becomes totally convincing with portrayals of muscle weakness, paralysis, pain, or tremors. Artfully applied makeup can render an SP pale or cyanotic or ashen. A fine spray of water onto skin that has been smoothed with vaseline results in perspiration. Rashes or hyperpigmentations, such as cafe-au-lait spots, can be applied. More sophisticated techniques can give an SP realistic-looking wounds in various stages of healing. Table 5.3 presents a partial list of dysfunctions that have been simulated. Behavioral characteristics that relate to a condition can also be mimicked. An SP with hyperthyroid may find it difficult to sit still during the interview and may complain of the "warm room". The patient with fatigue would find all movements and interactions an effort. The depressed patient may sign often, avoid eye contact, speak in a monotone, or

TABLE 5.2. Key to List of Available Simulations 1980–1981[a]

Interview—General
1. Ovarian cancer
2. Terminal cancer A
3. Terminal cancer B (metastatic carcinoma of brain and skeletal system)
4. Death and dying (fear of old age)
5. Schizophrenia A
6. Schizophrenia B
7. Schizophrenia C
8. Attempted suicide
9. Rape A
10. Rape B
11. Widowhood (grief and depression)
12. Drug abuse
13. Mastectomy
14. Alcoholic/arthritic A
15. Alcoholic/arthritic B
16. Vasectomy
17. Anorexia
18. Marital problems
19. Rash—birth control request
20. Manic
21. Unwed father—request for nerve pills
22. Angry patient—homicidal
23. Angry patient—fear of loss of function
24. The "worried well" patient

Interview—Families and couples
25. "Oddy" family
26. "Taylor" couple
27. "Lee" couple
28. "Theodore" couple
29. "Hunter" family
30. "Stewart" couple

[a]Simulated patient program: key to list of available simulations 1980–1981. Project for learning resources design. McMaster University, Faculty of Health Sciences. Hamilton, Ontario (mimeograph).

be weepy. An inability to concentrate may be exhibited by the SP. Stuttering or other speech problems may be portrayed. General appearance and behavioral characteristics coupled with anatomic and physiologic dysfunctions make the SP an ideal strategy for teaching physical assessment skills.

Realizing that it is artificial to separate history from physical when considering patient assessment, and that it is rare that an SP would be used only for the motor skills of the physical examination, this section nonetheless will focus solely on the physical examination. One skill that can be focused on is that of observation. Students may be required to describe what they see

**TABLE 5.3. Anatomic and Physiologic
Dysfunctions Portrayed by Simulated Patients**

Pain (partial list)
  Headache
  Neck
  Angina
  Backache
  Myalgias
  Claudication
  Abdominal
Tenderness
  With or without guarding
Sensory losses
Skin abnormalities
  Pallor
  Cyanosis
  Alterations of pigmentation
  Rashes
  Perspiration
  Wounds
Gait
  Parkinsonian
  Inebriated
Altered levels of consciousness
Memory loss
Coma
Seizures
Cranial nerve palsies
Muscle
  Hypertonicity
  Spasticity
  Weakness
  Paralysis
Tremors
Hyperkinesias
Dysmetria
Blindness
Pupil dilation
Collapsed lung
Hyperventilation
Aphasia
Affect
  Depression
  Inappropriate

using appropriate terminology. This may be in the context of normal or abnormal findings. The scope may be broad, such as general appearance, behavior, or gait. Or observations may be limited to a specific system or just to the systems related to the presenting problem. Applying knowledge of human anatomy to a specific body can be another use. Students can be asked to identify boney landmarks, major vessels, organs, and glands. Function may be assessed, discriminating normal from limited. If limited, the student may be asked to define the criteria used to evaluate the extent of the loss. The focus may be learning the actual motor skill necessary to conduct a physical examination. Students, when first learning these motor skills, often comment about feeling clumsy or awkward. "Where do I stand?" "How close should I be?" "Should I examine from the left or right side, with the patient lying or sitting?" This feeling of awkwardness is accentuated when they begin to use various tools—otoscope, ophthalmoscope, stethescope, reflex hammer.

Actual techniques can be practiced on the SP as many times as is necessary for the student to attain a certain level of ease. The SP is trained to expect this and will "reproduce" a physical finding as many times as it is examined. The focus may be an organizational one. The student may try different ways of organizing the elements of the examination to provide maximum efficiency, comfort, and safety for the patient. Another focus could be the verbal and nonverbal interactions between the student and as SP during the examination. Does the student look worried or preoccupied? How does the student respond to the SDSP's query of "is it normal?" after the examination of a part. Does the student provide reassurance and encouragement appropriately? The student may want to focus on the giving of instructions. It can be surprisingly difficult to give clear, concise instructions to enlist patient cooperation for the neurologic examination, for example. Manipulation of other factors such as a language barrier, a comprehension problem, fatigue, or age can make the challenge even greater.

The experience can be structured in ways similar to those discussed under interviewing. Instructor demonstration for the class may be used. In a small group setting, different students may complete different parts of the examination. For example, if the neurologic examination is being studied, one student may do the motor assessment, another the sensory, a third the cranial nerves, and so forth. Or all students may repeat the parts of the examination where a physical findings was identified. As with the interviewing, students can seek help from each other regarding approach, description, or assessment. It is important that only one person actually have "hands on" the SP at any given time. It takes great concentration to maintain a certain posture, affect, or functional loss. More than one simultaneous examiner is distracting and the quality of the simulation can be adversely affected.

Certain physical conditions are not possible to simulate, such as papilledema, enlarged liver, abnormal pulses. This situation can be handled in a variety of ways. The SP may hand the student examiner a 3" by 5" card stating the physical abnormality: liver dorn 5 cm with firm edge. Or, the instructor or the SP may give a verbal report at this point in the examination. At times, it may be appropriate to discuss these findings before the student begins the interaction with the SP. Student feedback about this limitation of the SP has been instructive. Properly handled, it has not been found to be disruptive to the *reality* of the situation.

The SP is trained to repeat the simulation as many times as necessary. Giving feedback is also part of the SP's role. Nonverbal and verbal feedback is given throughout the examination process, in keeping with the real patient's personality. A student who is too rough may get a verbal "ouch" or a side glance. A disorganized student may find the SP getting increasingly irritable and resistant to requests for position change. At the end of the learning session, the SP gives direct feedback to all students who participated in the examination. Again, remarks will be from the persepctive of how it felt to be that student's patient. "The worried look on your face when you listened to my heart made me anxious." "Your touch is very tentative and I wasn't sure if you really know what to do." "You always seemed aware of whether I was comfortable or not." "Your instructions were clear, but you didn't seem to notice how tired I was getting." These are the types of comments that an SP may make after the physical examination.

The role of the instructor remains basically the same as that during the interviewing session, that of a facilitator. Here, though, the instructor may take a more active role in demonstrating the skills, such as how to hold the otoscope and provide for the safety of the patient while examining the eardrum. Validation of findings both normal and abnormal are be provided by the instructor.

Response to the use of the SP for teaching physical assessment has been positive and enthusiastic. Maatsch[31] stated: "The limited evidence available suggests that the well-designed instructional and evaluative simulations may be more effective than clinical instruction based on real patients at the initial skill development stage." Table 5.4 presents a partial list of simulations that have been developed at the universities reportedly using this technique.

Simulated Patients and Nursing Education. Nursing faculty at Michigan State University used the SP as part of a four-stage sequence to help students learn assessment skills: (1) observation of a videotaped model demonstrating assessment, (2) supervised practice assessment with peers, (3) practice assessment with an SP, and (4) assessment of real patients.[32] Time with the SP was limited to 15 to 20 minutes, depending on the assigned task.

TABLE 5.4. Selected Simulations That Have Been Developed

Gastrointestinal
   Cessation of eating
   Overeating for which the patient wants slimming pills
   Epigastric pain
   Gastric ulcer
   Ulcer and depression
   Peptic ulcer
   Crohn's disease

Genitourinary
   Urinary tract infections
   Painless hematuria
   Venereal disease
   Vasectomy with complications
   Vasectomy failure with resultant pregnancy

Obstetrics and Gynecology
   Pelvic pain
   Abortion with resultant depression
   Sterility

Cardio-Respiratory
   Angina
   Pneumothorax
   Emphysema
   Heart failure

Neurology
   Dizziness
   Migraine
   Coma
   Subarachnoid hemorrhage
   Diabetic neuropathy
   Stroke
   Multiple sclerosis
   Polymyositis
   Parkinsons

Pain
   Sciatica
   Degenerating neck disc
   Low back pain
   Chronic low back pain

Internal Medicine
   Stress-related tension headache
   Sleeplessness
   Fatigue
   Hypo- and Hyperthyroidism
   Arthritis
   Diabetes
   Cholecystitis

Before actual contact with the SP, the student was given the basic information about the patient, that is, name, address, reason for the visit. A faculty member was available to provide assistance or to answer questions. After the activity, an assessment guide was completed and a problem list generated by the student. Students received feedback on the written work from the faculty. For the most part, students perceive this learning strategy as helpful. Their comments point to the fact that the goals for the learning experience were met.

The SP's ability to recall historical facts, portray a personality with all the congruent reactions, and assume the behavioral and physical characteristics of the actual patient, makes this a valuable teaching strategy for learning the arts, science, and mechanics of health assessment in nursing. It is also a useful strategy for teaching problem-solving skills.

Additionally, the use of an SP is an excellent strategy for helping nursing students learn a systematic approach to the assessment of patient problems. It is one thing to learn the steps of problem solving in class, but it is yet another to incorporate them into an interaction with a real patient. Much has been written about the gap between a students' classroom learning and their application in the clinical setting. With the SP, the student can practice this application. One way to accomplish this is to have the student assess the SP in a small group setting. In the same manner as described, one student can begin the assessment requesting help from peers and faculty as necessary. Or students may take turns. Whichever form is used, the focus of the experience is the cognitive process. Any any time during the interview or physical examination the student may be stopped and asked one of the following questions:

What are you thinking now?
What hypotheses have you generated?
What information do you have that supports your hypotheses?
What additional information do you need?

In this way, the cognitive processes of the student can be explored as attempts are made to apply knowledge to a clinical situation. Common student difficulties can be identified. For example, frequently students do not thoroughly explore the patient's definition of a word. The patient may complain of "dizziness," which may mean "faint" to one patient and vertigo to another. "Constipation" may mean "only once a day" to a mother of a new baby and "no bowel movement for five days" to another mother. Accurately defining what terms mean to the patient is important for making an accurate assessment.

Closely related to this is accepting a patient's own diagnosis without obtaining enough information to substantiate or refute it. Taking such statements as "I'm allergic to penicillin" or "I have migraine headaches" at face value is a common student error. All students struggle with how much information to obtain and in what areas to pursue more data. For example, if a patient is complaining of a poor appetitie or fatigue, what questions need to be asked and what parts of the physical examination need to be done? Experience with an SP can address all these issues effectively. The focus of the experience can be the data-gathering process, or it can be extended to "making the assessment." The student can be required to state the assessment with a supportive summary of historical and physical findings. The consideration here is whether or not the student had adequate and accurate data to support the assessment. If not, where is the problem? Perhaps there is a knowledge gap, or it may be that the data has been interpreted incorrectly. The focus of the experience can be extended further to nursing management. When the whole process is completed, another common student problem may become apparent. Often, students fall into the habit of addressing management issues before the assessment has been made. A student may lanuch into teaching during data gathering. The problem is that time may be spent on an aspect of patient management that in the final assessment, assumes a lesser priority. For example, a student may launch into a five-minute teaching intervention regarding foot hygiene early in the interview of a diabetic patient, only to discover later that the patient is giving his insulin incorrectly. Top priority should be spending time on proper administration of insulin. Foot hygiene would be part of the follow-up plan.

Through experience with an SP, the student can learn the importance of the systematic approach, of making assessments and establishing priorities before engaging in management of care. Other nursing process issues can be addressed through the following sample questions:

What evidence do you have that the patient understands _____?
   (specifics to be chosen)
In what ways did you include the patient in the management plan?
Did you identify specifics in the patient's situation (for example, values, family supports, home situation, finances) that will support or interfere with compliance?

The questions selected on management will depend on a variety of factors, such as level of the student and the clinical setting presented.

Besides examining elements of the cognitive process, the SP can be used to explore the affective domain. The student can be stopped at any time during the interaction with the SP and be asked "What are you feeling?" How feelings impact on the problem-solving process can be the focus of the activity. A student, for example, may feel very uncomfortable with the issue of child abuse, and fail to identify that a history does not support the type of injury presenting. The student may avoid asking about physical signs, such as excessive bruising, or about disciplinary practices. This aspect of nurse–patient interactions cannot be as effectively presented in the lecture format. Time constraints and the demands of patient needs usually prohibit this focus of learning in the clinical laboratory. Use of the SP can help a student, in a nonpressured setting, identify feelings and begin to see the effect they have on the problem-solving process.

Another way an SP may be used is as a stimulus for discussion. After an experience with an SP, class members may focus on management issues. What is the best plan for this patient in view of what we know about alternative nursing interventions and the patient's home situation? A theory, such as crisis theory, may be applied to the patient situation.[33] Or the focus may be the different roles of team members who are involved in patient care. It may be a springboard for discussion of ethical issues. Because all class members have shared the same "patient experience," participation in subsequent discussions tends to be active.

Simulated Patient and Evaluation.   The SP is an excellent evaluative tool when clinical skills are being tested. Dissatisfaction with use of multiple choice, true/false, or essay exams for the testing of clinical skills has been expressed in evaluation literature, as well as by medical and nursing educators alike. The performance of nurses as they relate directly with patients is perhaps the most important aspect of their professional behavior. Use of the SP allows evaluation of this major component of nursing. An actual case that is representative of the course content may be chosen for the basis of the SP use. The level of the student to be tested will determine the complexity of the case. Specific criteria for evaluation need to be developed. Because the SP's rendition is infinitely repeatable, all students are evaluated in the same patient situation. The evaluation can be structured to focus on specific student behaviors during one patient interaction. Examples are shown in Table 5.5. Another option is to structure the situation so that the student "cares for the patient over time." One encounter could be day one of a hospitalization and a second encounter just before discharge. This latter form may be used to evaluate a student's ability to assess and plan nursing management during different stages of a patient's illness. A number of reports in the literature describe and support this use of the SP.

Medical students rotating through a family practice clerkship at Southern Illinois University were evaluated at the completion of the family practice experience.[34] Simulated Patients were scripted with relatively straightforward medical problems. Students were aware that the patients were simulat-

**TABLE 5.5. Evaluation of Student Behaviors Using the Simulated
Patient**

Ability to obtain historical data
Ability to assess reliability of data and its relevance to the problem
Interviewing skills
Physical examination skills
Organization
Terminology
Ability to identify patient problems
Inclusion of patient in management plan
Ability to formulate realistic, beneficial management plan
Ability to evaluate outcomes
Ability to evaluate self

ed. At the beginning of the session the student was given a brief chart and allowed a few minutes to review it and ask questions of the faculty present. They were then instructed to interview the patient and obtain a history. Twenty minutes was allotted. The interview was videotaped for later discussion.

Upon completion of the interview, the student discussed it with the faculty member and identified parts of the physical examination that would be appropriate. The faculty supplied the physical findings verbally, including the results of any tests about which the student inquired. The student then went back to the patient and explained the management plan. The faculty evaluator who had observed the student's interaction with the SP completed a History Check Sheet, an Interview Assessment and rating sheets for the student's physical examination, and generated a problem list and management plan. These, plus an SP feedback form were reviewed with the student. Students also had the opportunity to review the video with the faculty.

After all the students completed the examination, they met and discussed the case, so it became a valuable learning experience for several students. The SP technique was so successful that it was extended to the undergraduate teaching program in which SPs were used in the behavioral science curriculum to teach students how to deal with different personality types presenting with health problems.

A number of medical programs in the United States and Cananda use SP for evaluation purposes.[35,36,37] Barrows and Tamblyn[38] designed an alternative method for clinical skills evaluation called a self-assessment unit. It allows the student to perfrom self-evaluation without the need for a faculty observer. The SP also was used as a portion of the 1970 Certification Examination of the College of Family Physicians of Canada to assess the performance of the candidates.[39]

Besides evaluation of students or physicians, the use of an SP is also useful for standardization of evaluators. Evaluators observe a student conducting a visit with an SP and then individually evaluate the student. Then the evaluators discuss how and why they evaluated the student as they did. This is very useful for identifying expectations of students—faculty agreement as well as areas of conflict. Faculty at the University of Connecticut used the SP in this way. The total faculty, undergraduate and graduate, observed a student–SP interaction that included history taking and physical examination. Each faculty member completed an evaluation form rating the student: junior faculty as if it were a junior student, senior faculty as if it were a senior student, and likewise for graduate faculty. General discussion followed. It provided an excellent vehicle for stimulating open discussion of expectations of students' assessment skills at the three levels. This experience gave faculty insight into two areas of evaluation that needed addressing: blurring of student expectations within levels and between levels, and varied perceptions of student behavior. Use of the SP provided an opportunity for faculty to see and understand these two problem areas and to look at ways to handle them.

Use of the Simulated Patient in Graduate and Undergraduate Education.
All of the described uses of the SP are equally suited to graduate and undergraduate learning. The same SP can be used for learning on these different levels. What would distinguish the two would be the focus of the learning experience or the level of the objectives and the expectation of the student. For example, if interviewing is the focus of learning, the undergraduate level student may be learning introduction of self, explanation of the student nursing role, organization, and phrasing of questions. The focus of the graduate student may be on the more affective elements of the interviewing process. For example, the challenge may be to help the patient identify his feelings. The student may attempt this by carefully observing nonverbal behavior and reflecting these observations back to the patient. On either the graduate or undergraduate level, if one interviewing approach does not seem successful, the student can stop, rethink, and then try another approach.

Summary.   The SP as a teaching strategy has many uses in nursing ranging from the practice of skills to evaluation. The advantages of this strategy are many. Students experience a real situation without risk to an actual patient. There is no need to worry about saying or doing something to endanger the patient. The student does not have to feel embarrassed or threatened by not knowing something in the presence of an actual patient. The self-esteem of students is enhanced when fewer initial blunders are made on real patients. With the SP, a variety of interpersonal skills or approaches to the physical assessment can be practiced until the student gains ease and a certain comfort level or mastery. There is no time restriction. Students can take as long as necessary to conduct an interview and physical assessment.

Availability is another advantage. Faculty do not have to depend on patient cases available at the time of the clinical laboratory activities. The use of an SP can be planned well in advance. This provides time for specific objectives to be developed, as well as criteria for a successful learning experience. Cases that are difficult to obtain can be simulated. There are other times when a student would gain by experience with a sensitive problem, such as infertility, but because of patient needs at the time, faculty would be reluctant to make the assignment. An SP can make the situation available to all students.

Another advantage is repeatability. Every student sees the same signs and symptoms. The variable is the student, whether it be in skill level, that is, ability to elicit a sign, or in observational acuity, that is, ability to see the sign. The SP can be examined any numbers of times and the symptoms and signs remain constant.

Use of the SP also affords controllability. Simple or complex situations can be chosen for simulation. The setting can be chosen and staged—inpatient or outpatient. The intensity of the situation can be controlled. A weepy patient can be instructed to exhibit only a few sniffles for the beginning student, and to weep uncontrollably for the advanced student. A loquacious patient can be tuned up to make a challenging control situation for the interviewing student, or tuned down to make the situation more easily managed. The amount of information given to the student can also be contolled. The SP may be "reluctant" to answer questions when they contain many medical terms. The SP may not offer any information about a strong family history of cancer and how fearful that makes her, unless specifically asked to do so. These elements can be graduated according to student levels and needs.

It is a highly adaptable learning strategy. The SP can be used individually, in small groups, or in a large classroom setting. The same simulation can be used for different levels of students, undergraduate through graduate. At any time during the use of the SP, the process can be interrupted for discussion of problems or findings. This can occur in the presence of the SP. When necessary, the process can be stopped so outside resources can be consulted, and then continued at a later date when the information has been found. Because the case of the real patient is known, it is possible to follow the problem through to the end. This is accomplished by simulating the patient at one stage of the problem and then for the same problem at a later stage.

Immediate feedback is available to the student after an interaction with a SP. The feedback is honest, direct, and more useful to the student than the usually protective feedback of real patients. Feedback from a SP is also less anxiety-provoking to the student because no harm is done to a real patient. The SP who is perceptive, articulate, and sensitive can assist a student to see shortcomings and possibilities for improvement without feeling threatened.

The main advantage is that the focus can be *learning*. Students have an opportunity to apply skills and knowledge to a clinical situation without the pressure of real patient needs.

There are also disadvantages to the SP as a learning strategy. All physical findings cannot be simulated, and alternative ways of informing the student about them may prove distracting. Students may not take the experience with the SP seriously because they are not dealing with a real patient. Occasionally students miss the point of certain SP behaviors. A student who asked too many personal questions too early in the interview with an adolescent, complained to the faculty person afterwards. "Next time, you should simulate a patient who talks more." This student attributed the SP's reticence to other factors, and did not make the connection that the silence was in response to poor interviewing skills. Because the focus of the learning is process as well as content, this strategy takes more time in the classroom or clinical setting.

Steps in Simulating the Patient.   The first step is selection of an individual who would make a good simulated patient. There are a number of attributes that should be looked for when interviewing candidates. The person should have an ability to remember a history and to ad lib appropriately when the "unexpected question" is asked by the student. The person should be able to portray the personality and emotional and physical characteristics of the real patient. This takes good concentration powers as well as physical stamina. Good general health is necessary. Current or past experience with the patient problem that is to be simulated eliminates that candidate for that simulation. A similar personal situation, direct or indirect, for example, a mother-in-law with the same condition or experience with the problem, may be personally difficult for the candidate. Although the candidate may deny that it would be difficult to portray the problem, experience has shown that attempting the simulation often recalls forgotten feelings and conflicts.

An ability to separate the candidates own feelings from those of the simulated patient is necessary. The individual must also be able to identify student behaviors that facilitate or impede the client–nurse relationship. Being able to sensitively give this feedback to the student is also important.

There are practical aspects, such as availability, that also need to be explored. The person must be available during the hours that the faculty member is most likely to need him or her. If the candidate is a parent responsible for child care, reliable babysitting arrangements must be possible. Having their own transportation or access to good public transportation is also a consideration. Experience has shown that candidates who need the extra money tend to be the SPs who are most available.

Some educational programs have used actors and actresses, professional as well as student. As a group, they have had mixed reviews. Faculty have praised them for their ability to communicate the real patient. On the other hand, some faculty have commented that the actors and actresses tend to get so involved with their technique that they forget to respond as the student's patient. Consequently, their ability to give useful feedback to the student is compromised. Students from other departments within the university have been used. The only problem special to this group is availability. Class schedules may conflict. If needed in the nursing program for evaluative purposes, it tends to be at the same time they are facing midterms or finals. The student is less available when you may need the SP most. Most faculty experienced with using this teaching strategy agree that health professionals are to be avoided. They tend to bring their own biases to the situation and may be too easy or too difficult on the student.

Having chosen the person for the simulation, the next step is the training. This should be done by someone familiar with the actual patient to be simulated, some familiar with the history, physical and emotional characteristics, and personality of the patient. Ideally this would stem from face-to-face contact in a care-giving capacity. Another way to accomplish this is to review the patient's record and talk with care-givers.

The simulator tells the SP about the patient. While hearing the description, the SP writes notes that will help with recall. The simulator responds to any questions the SP has about the case. The questions may be for additional history or for better understanding of what it would be like to be that patient having that procedure. The SP may never have experienced the particular patient setting, and may need a description of it. Because it is impossible to know all the facts about another individual, there will be gaps that are not critical to the simulation. Perhaps the nutritional history of the real patient has no special meaning to the problem. In this situation, the SP's own nutritional history can be used. The same holds true for other historical data. If the SP feels uncomfortable using his or her own history, something appropriate and familiar can be made up. This initial sessions usually takes one hour. At the end, the SP is advised to go home and think about what it would be like to be this patient. Questions that come up should be recorded and brought to the next session.

At the second session, the SP's questions are answered and further augmentation is completed. The next skill that needs to be learned is portrayal of physical findings. The simulator demonstrates the finding, such as a posture or gait or tremor, and the SP practices until the finding can be replicated. Then the simulator "examines" the SP so the SP learns how to maintain the findings during a phsyical examination. This is also the way to check the SP's ability to mimic the physical finding. This aspect takes one to two hours.

The "dry run" is an important element of the training of an SP. A faculty or health professional or student experienced with the SP strategy, completes a history and physical examination on the SP. It gives the SP a chance to practice. It is also a way to check the "realistic" quality of the simulation. The SP may forget to maintain a characteristic style of verbal response throughout the whole encounter. An unanticipated question may catch the SP off guard. Being able to identify the problems and correct them ahead of time will greatly improve the quality of the SP as a teaching strategy. Persons who are new to the concept of the SP may need more than one dry run. This need decreases significantly with experience.

The SP is now ready for use in the classroom or laboratory setting. The faculty in charge of the learning experience is responsible for briefing the SP. The objectives of the learning experience are reviewed. These may relate to interviewing skills, physical assessment skills, problem solving, and so forth. The SP is apprised of student capabilities. "This is their first experience interviewing and they will probably be quite anxious." Or, "These students are near completion of the cardiovascular unit and should be organized and efficient in completing your assessment." If the students have particular problem areas that the simulation addresses, the SP is told of these. Having this knowledge allows the SP to give more useful feedback to the students. The format to be used is reviewed. For example, the format may be a small group and each student will individually interview or examine the SP. As necessary, the simulation is reviewed. This may be a last minute test of a physical finding, such as muscle weakness, or answering a question about the history.

Once the students have completed their interaction with the SP and their discussion, the SP gives feedback to the students. Having been given a few minutes to "recover" from portraying the patient, the SP focuses on articulating to each student what he or she felt like to be the student's patient. The parameters of this feedback were presented earlier in this chapter. After the feedback, the faculty and SP go to an area away from the students for the debriefing. During the debriefing, the SP received feedback on the quality of the simulation. Strong points, such as style or response to the different students, are reinforced. Suggestions for improvement are made if there were any problems. It is also a time for the SP to mention any areas that proved difficult, or any questions that arose. The faculty should review with the SP how the simulation met the objectives for the session. The debriefing is a very necessary and important part of the SP training.

Sample Case for Simulation

Professor Rolli, a faculty member in a university school of nursing, was responsible for teaching the graduate client assessment course. Classes were limited to eight students. Course content included interviewing, history-taking, and examination of all body systems. For each system, students were responsible for knowing relevant history questions, anatomy and physiology, and techniques used to conduct the physical assessment. Teaching strategies included lecture, demonstration, role-playing, and pairing of students to examine each other. Because the neurologic system is complex and includes a number of other systems (for example, eye, skin), it was placed at the end of the course and was allotted two consecutive three-hour classes. The neurologic examination is also one that includes a variety of maneuvers that need to be organized, and, therefore, it requires the use of several instruments and necessitates the cooperation of a client to accomplish it. Consequently, Professor Rolli decided to use an SP as a teaching strategy. The first class was a lecture and demonstration of the neurologic assessment. Students were assigned to practice the different elements of the examination and to prepare to interview and examine a "patient" who had a diagnosis of multiple sclerosis in the following class.

Unknown to the class was the fact that the "patient" was an SP. The SP had been trained by Professor Rolli. Because it was the first time this strategy had been used in the school of nursing, the first step was to find an individual who was interested, motivated, and capable. The "real" patient was a 48-year-old female, so the SP needed to be female and between 20 and 60 years of age. Phone calls were made to the drama school, the Women's Health Center, and to local residents. Secretaries in the school of nursing were approached to determine if they knew anyone who might be interested. It took many calls, many explanations, and nearly three weeks before an interested and available candidate was located. She was interviewed, and besides being in good health and having had no previous experience with the problem, she had many of the personal characteristics that contribute to a good SP. Her husband was a graduate student at the university. She was taking one night course. They had one young child, good babysitting arrangements, transportation, and were in need of extra money. She liked the concept of the SP and Professor Rolli thought that she would be a good one. The first training session was arranged. The agreed upon salary was $5 per hour, including training time.

The first session took about 90 minutes. Professor Rolli had personally cared for the patient and could accurately describe personality and emotional responses as well as relate historic and physical data. The SP had many questions about the social situation of the family and about what certain hospital procedures, such as a myelogram, were like. At the end of the session, the SP was asked to think about what it would be like to be this particular woman with multiple sclerosis and a young family. She also was to document any questions that she thought of that related to the case or to her role as the SP.

The second session was held the following week. History was reviewed and more details were added. For such areas as diet history and her family of origin, the SP was to use her own history. The training then turned to the physical findings. First, Professor Rolli described each finding and explained what caused it. Then she demonstrated it. For example, the patient had a characteristic gait. Then the SP was "examined" so she would know the type of maneuvers that would be done. It was then her turn to mimic the physical findings and be examined. This session took 90 minutes.

The next week was the dry run. Another faculty who was knowledgeable about neurologic assessment interviewed and examined the SP as if it were a real client visit. The SP received feedback on her abilities. She lost concentration once and giggled nervously. She had trouble being weak on the right side (arm and leg) throughout the examination. She was too quick to "help" the examiner during a part of the examination. The real patient would have needed more instructions before she could have completed it. The other elements—the personality portrayal, affect, posture, tremors—were well done.

The SP was surprised at the amount of concentration that was required. She also was concerned about the unexpected questions that might be posed by a student. To assist her, more possible questions were given to her. She was also reassured that as she became more comfortable in the role, the questions would be less threatening. At this time, how to give feedback was reviewed. The SP was quick to understand its purpose and the type of feedback she was to give. Neither the SP nor the Professor felt the need for another dry run. The SP was to write the case in her own words and this would be her reference. The write-up was as follows:

Mary Dodd

The "patient" was a 48-year-old woman with multiple sclerosis who we called Mary Dodd. She was married and the mother of three children, two boys age 27 and 14, and one girl age 17. Her disease was diagnosed 11 years ago and since that time the synptoms have gotten progressively worse.

Her symptoms started with tingling in the hands. She now complains of exhaustion, generalized weakness, and numbness of the bottom of her feet up to her knees. Bad weather causes a general increase in symptoms. She once had a blind spot in one eye that has since gone away. She wears glasses for distance but other than that has no vision problems. She had bells palsy when she was 28 years old.

Her family history includes a father, who died of amyotrophic lateral sclerosis (ALS) when Mary was a young girl. She has an aunt who is an epileptic. Her youngest son had Down's Syndrome. He also had a thyroid problem that had been corrected and has resulted in more activity on his part.

Miscellaneous:

She has slight drooping on left side of face due to bells palsy.

She has frequent urination and must take pills when she goes out to control problem.

Her fingers are stiff in the morning and she has problems with fine motor coordination.

Her response to physical testing is as follows:

"Buzz test": did not feel buzz from knees down.

Position test: was not able to distinguish the position of toes but was able to distinguish hands.

Cotton Test: did not feel from knees down.

Sharp or dull: could distinguish.

Mental status: could not remember three objects in 5-minute time.

Reflex test on foot: toes curled up instead of down.

Before entering the classroom, the SP was briefed. She was told that these were graduate nursing students who should have skills in interviewing and making her comfortable. Their previous content regarding the neurologic examination was reviewed and she was told that they had limited supervised practice and could be expected to be somewhat awkward. The objectives of the learning experience were:

Interview a patient with a neurologic problem using the problem-based approach.

Conduct a physical examination.

Summarize the case ending with the nursing assessment.

The format was to be a small group, one student interviewing or examining at a time, with opportunities for *time out*. A last minute review of physical findings was conducted. The SP was properly "weak" and had good "tremors." Her questions were answered.

The students were told that the setting was a primary care office. A nurse would be interviewing and examining a new patient. The patient was a 48-year-old woman with a history of multiple sclerosis who had just moved to the vicinity from another state. The patient wanted to establish her health care.

The SP was then brought into the "the office". The class went smoothly. It was interesting to note how quickly the students assumed that the patient was real. They became more attentive and concerned about the woman, her history, and her comfort as she was questioned and examined. There were a number of time outs to obtain help from peers. During this time, the SP would gaze in a direction opposite the students to maintain her concentration. Her physical findings were so convincing that each student wanted and was able to examine her. At the end, one student presented the case and the assessment.

The SP was able during the presentation to recover and collect her thoughts about feedback. She then gave sensitive, helpful feedback to each student. After this, the SP and professor went into an office for debriefing. "How she did" was discussed. Her ability to maintain concentration for the whole session was praised. Her history was accurate, except for confusing dates of birth of her children. They didn't correlate with the ages! The unexpected questions she had handled well and in keeping with the real case. Her physical dysfunctions were excellent. The SP expressed exhaustion and was surprised at how much energy it required to portray the patient and be thinking about the students' behavior and style. She had a few questions about the history, related to not knowing what some of the tests were that the students had asked her about. The professor then discussed how the SP had helped in meeting the objectives for the learning session.

The students were quite excited about the activity. The patient did seem "real" and yet they didn't have anxiety about harming or inconveniencing a real patient. They liked having the opportunity to "put it all together" while still having the support of peers and instructor. They commented that they approached the interviewing and examination of the SP in a much more serious fashion than when they practiced on each other.

Notes

1. Kramer, M., Holaday, B., & Hoeffer, B. The teaching of nursing research—part II: A literature review of teaching strategies. *Nurse Educator*, 1981, 6 (2), 30–37.

2. McKenzie, L. Simulation games and adult education. *Adult Leadership*, 1974, 22 (5), 293–295.

3. Erickson, E. H., & Borgmeyer, S. V. Simulated decision-making experience via case analysis. *Journal of Nursing Administration*, 1979, 9 (5), 10–15.

4. Bailey, J. T., & Claus, K. E. *Decision making in nursing, tools for change*. St. Louis: C. V. Mosby, 1975.

5. Corbett, N. A., & Beveridge, P. Simulation as a tool for learning. *Topics in Clinical Nursing*, 1982, 4 (3), 58–67.

6. Barrows, H. S., & Tamblyn, R. M. *Problem-based learning: An approach to medical education*. New York: Springer Publishing Company, 1980.

7. Fibison-Boniface, W. J., & Rideout, E. *Problem based learning unit in primary care nursing no. PCP1*. Prepared for Educational Program for Nurses in Primary Care Program. Hamilton, Ontario: McMaster University, 1977.

8. deTornyay, R. Measuring problem-solving skills by means of the simulated clinical nursing problem test. *Journal of Nursing Education*, 1968, 7 (3), 3–8, 34, 35.

9. Page, G. G. Written simulation in nursing. *Journal of Nursing Education*, 1978, 17 (4), 28–32.

10. Taylor, A. P. Clinical simulations in nursing. *Nursing Times*, 1980, 76 (28), 1217–1218.

11. Keller, M. L., & MacCormick, K. N. From graduate students to faculty: A simulation. *Nursing Outlook*, 1980, 28 (5), 305–307.

12. Gerrard, B. A., & Buzzell, E. M. *Behavioral test of interpersonal skills for health professionals*. Reston, Virginia: Reston Publishing Company, 1979.

13. Crancer, J., & Maury-Hess, S. Games: An alternative to pedagogical instruction. *Journal of Nursing Education*, 1980, 19 (3), 45–52.

14. Davidhizar, R. E. Use of simulation games in teaching psychiatric nursing. *Journal of Nursing Education*, 1977, 16 (5), 9–12.

15. Baldwin, E. Senior center experience of a student nurse. *Journal of Gerontological Nursing*, 1979, 5 (2), 22–24.

16. The Ohio Department of Mental Health and Mental Retardation. *Humanization game*. *Motive*, Columbus, Ohio.

17. Chaisson, G. M. Life-cycle: A social-simulation game to improve attitudes and responses to the elderly. *Journal of Gerontological Nursing*, 1980, 6 (10), 587–592.

18. Ibid, p. 592.

19. Barrows, H. S. *Simulated patients*. Springfield, Illinois: C. C. Thomas, 1971.

20. Engel, I. M., Resnick, P. J., & Levine, S. B. The use of programmed patients and videotape in teaching medical students to take a sexual history. *Journal of Medical Education,* 1976, *51* (5), 425–427.

21. Hannay, D. R. Teaching interviewing with simulated patients. *Medical Education,* 1980, *14* (4), 246–248.

22. Jewett, L. S., Greenberg, L. W., Champion, L. A., Gluck, R. S., Leikin, S. L. Altieri, M. F., & Lipnick, R. N. The teaching of crisis counseling skills to pediatric residents: A one-year study. *Pediatrics,* 1982, *70* (6), 907–911.

23. Lincoln, R., Layton, J., & Holdman, H. Using simulated patients to teach assessment. *Nursing Outlook,* 1978, *26* (5), 316–320.

24. Maguire, G. P., Clark, D., & Jolley, B. An experimental comparison of three courses in history-taking skills for medical students. *Medical Education,* 1977, 11 (3), 175–182.

25. Kerr, M. G., Templeton, A. A., & Purboosingh, J. Simulated patients as a learning resource in the study of reproductive medicine. *Medical Education,* 1977, *11* (6), 374–376.

26. Engel, I. M., Resnick, P. J., & Levine, S. B. The use of programmed patients and videotape in teaching medical students to take a sexual history. *Journal of Medical Education,* 1976, *51* (5), 425–427.

27. Jewett, L. S., Greenberg, L. W., Champion, L. A., Gluck, R. S., Leikin, S. L., Altieri, M. F., & Lipnick, R. N. The teaching of crisis counseling skills to pediatric residents: A one-year study. *Pediatrics,* 1982, *70* (6), 907–911.

28. Jason, H., Kagan, N., Werner, A., Elstein, A. S., & Thomas, J. B. New approaches to teaching basic interview skills to medical students. *American Journal of Psychiatry,* 1971, *127* (10), 1404.

29. Maguire, P. The use of patient simulation in training medical students in history-taking skills. *Medical and Biological Illustration,* 1976, *26* (2), 91–93.

30. Neufeld, V. R., & Barrows, H. S. The McMaster philosophy: An approach to medical education. *Journal of Medical Education,* 1974, *49* (11), 1040–1050.

31. Maatsch, J. *A study of simulation technology in medical education: Main paper.* East Lansing, Michigan: Office of Medical Education, Research and Development, Michigan State University, 1977, p. 10 (Mimeograph).

32. Lincoln, R., Layton, J., & Holdman, H. Using simulated patients to teach assessment. *Nursing Outlook,* 1978, *26* (5), 316–320.

33. Infante, M. S. (Ed.). *Crisis theory: A framework for nursing practice.* Reston, Virginia: Reston Publishing Company, 1982.

34. Coggan, P. G., Knight, P. K., & Davis, P. D. Evaluating students in family medicine using simulated patients. *Journal of Family Practice*, 1980, *10* (2), 259–265.

35. Holmes, F. F., Baber, L. H., Torian, E. C. Measuring clinical competence of medical students. *Medical Education*, 1978, *12* (5), 364–368.

36. Sanson-Fisher, R. W., & Poole, A. D. Simulated patients and the assessment of medical students' interpersonal skills. *Medical Education*, 1980, *14* (4), 249–253.

37. Barrows, H. S. Simulated patients in medical teaching. *Canadian Medical Association Journal*, 1968, *98* (14), 674–676.

38. Barrows, H. S., & Tamblyn, R. M. Self-assessment units. *Journal of Medical Education*, 1976, *51* (4), 334–336.

39. Lamont, C. T., & Hennen, B. K. The use of simulated patients in a certification examination in family medicine. *Journal of Medical Education*, 1972, *47* (10), 789–795.

Bibliography

Anderson, K. K., & Meyer, T. C. The use of instructor-patients to teach physical examination techniques. *Journal of Medical Education*, 1978, 53 (10), 831–836.

Barrows, H. S., & Abrahamson, S. The programmed patient: A technique for appraising student performance in clinical neurology. *Journal of Medical Education*, 1964, 39 (8), 802–805.

Barrows, H. S., & Tamblyn, R. M. An evaluation of problem-based learning in small groups utilizing a simulated patient. *Journal of Medical Education*, 1976, 51 (1), 52–54.

Boocock, S. S. (Ed.). *Simulation games in learning*. Beverly Hills, California: Sage Publishers, 1968.

Clark, C. C. Simulation gaming: A new teaching strategy in nursing education. *Nurse Educator*, 1976, 1 (4), 4–9.

Cooper, S. S. Methods of teaching—revisited games and simulation. *Journal of Continuing Education in Nursing*, 1979, 10 (5), 14, 47–48.

Corbett, N. A., & Beveridge, P. *Clinical simulations in nursing practice*. Philadelphia: W. B. Saunders Co., 1980.

Davidhizar, R. E. Use of the simulation games in teaching psychiatric nursing. *Journal of Nursing Education*, 1977, 16 (5), 9–12.

Ehlinger, J., Miller, A. G., Farrand, L. A., & Wexzemer, W. L. A simulated patient encounter for the family nurse practitioner. *Journal of Nursing Education*, 1979, 18 (5), 5–15.

Farrell, M., Haley, M., & Magnasco, J. Teaching interpersonal skills. *Nursing Outlook*, 1977, 25 (5), 322–325.

Freer, C. B. Videotape recording in the assessment of the history-taking skills of medical students. *Medical Education*, 1978, *12* (4), 360–363.

Jeffers, J. M., & Christensen, M. G. Using simulation to facilitate the acquisition of clinical observational skills. *Journal of Nursing Education*, 1979, *18* (6), 29–32.

Laszlo, S. S., & McKenzie, J. L. The use of a simulation game in training hospital staff about patient rights. *Journal of Continuing Education in Nursing*, 1979, 10 (5), 30–36.

Lehrer, S. S. The professional patient session as a technique for teaching the gynecological examination to nurse practitioner students. *Journal of Nursing Education*, 1980, *19* (5), 39–47.

Livingstone, R. A., & Ostrow, D. N. Professional patient-instructors in the teaching of the pelvic exam. *American Journal of Obstetrics and Gynecology*, 1978, *132* (1), 64–67.

Lowe, J. Games and simulations in nurse education. *Nursing Mirror*, 1975, *141* (23), 68–69.

Nafulin, D. H., & Andrew, B. J. The effects of patient simulations on actors. *Journal of Medical Education*, 1975, *50* (1), 87–89.

Owen, A., & Underwood, P. Videotape and simulated patients. *Medical Journal of Australia*, 1980, *1* (9), 437–440.

Rottet, S. M. Gaming as a learning strategy. *Journal of Continuing Education in Nursing*, 1974, *5* (6), 22–25.

Stillman, P. A., Levinson, M. D., Rugill, J., & Sabers, D. An objective method of assessing physical examination skills of nurse practitioners. *Journal of Nursing Education*, 1979, *18* (3), 31–32.

Wolf, M. S., & Coggins, C. C. A workshop for development of simulation games in nursing. *Journal of Continuing Education in Nursing*, 1981, *12* (3), 31–34.

Yantzie, N. Help: Simulated disaster game. *The Canadian Nurse*, 1980, *76* (6), 33–36.

CHAPTER 6

Consideration of Participants Involved in the Process of Clinical Teaching

The process of clinical teaching is exceedingly complex. All the preceding considerations attest to the many considerations to be made by the nurse educator with responsibilities for clinical teaching. In fact, the totality of the role demands of the nurse faculty member as it relates to clinical teaching can be overwhelming to the novice teacher. And, admittedly, despite the numerous facets of the discussion, the analysis of the use of the clinical laboratory in nursing education has been limited to educational concerns, that is, the process of teaching and learning for practice in a clinical setting. A thorough exploration of this type is needed to serve as a point of reference as to the essence of a clinical laboratory and the intended use of it.

However, an important factor that contributes to the complexity of clinical teaching is the many persons involved in the process. Understanding the perspective of each of these groups of persons is of the utmost importance if the availability, accessibility, and needed usage of clinical settings is to be afforded and maintained. The goals of each group are essentially the same—the provision of quality nursing care. The roles of each are complementary: the role of the nurse educator is to produce quality practitioners who will render quality nursing care; the role of the student is to become a quality practitioner of nursing; the role of current practitioners of nursing is to model a quality practitioner and deliver quality care; and the role of administrators of educational programs and nursing service is to facilitate the educational and service goals of the nurses within their purview. Equally important is the client or consumer of the care rendered.

All are involved in the process of caring and all are involved in the process of educating students to become caregivers. An appropriate role exists for each. Without attention to these roles, especially as they have evolved in current day situations, there is interference with the educational process. The result is that the nurse educator faces constraints on the learning process in clinical settings that could have negative, lasting outcomes for the learner. The student suffers, but the client is ultimately the recipient of these shortcomings. With some cognizance of the needs, immediate goals, and appropriate roles of each group, the teaching and learning in clinical settings could be enhanced.

The following discussion examines four groups of persons participating in the process of clinical instruction: learners, teachers, clients, and the administrators of educational and clinical agencies along with their nursing staff.

Needs of the Learner in Clinical Laboratory

The nursing student, or the learner, expects to have ample opportunity to use the clinical laboratory for the purpose of practicing the application of theory to practice. The learner needs to use varied settings, at varied times, for specific purposes to be afforded the set of experiences basic to *becoming* a nurse. This learner needs to be actively involved in the student-related and other-related elements presented earlier. Reilly[1] describes the student's purpose for being in clinical practice in a somewhat different manner. She states that clinical field practice affords students the opportunity to relate theory to practice, develop their own theory of practice, learn to learn, handle ambiguity, think like a professional, and accept personal causation (accountability). In short, the selected use of the lclinical laboratory is essential to taking on the characteristics of the practicing nurse.

Yet, the costs of professional education are rising. Students are paying a high price for learning. Laboratory sessions are inherently expensive. But faculty strive to keep costs within limits through the most efficient use of the clinical laboratory. That involves using the clinical laboratory only when client contact is needed, when goals are clear in the mind of the learners, and when appropriate opportunities to apply the theory being studied to practice have been selected. Also, each hour spent by the learner in the clinical laboratory should be devoted to learning, that is, the transfer of theory to practice. To do otherwise and to use credit time for the repetition of tasks, for activities that the learner has not learned, or for working vaguely stated objectives results in a misuse of tuition monies and the time of all involved. Moreover, freeing the learner from the demands of tasks, the responsibility for care, and adherence to the routine of a service agency is expected to result in both the time, inclination, and freedom to learn. Learners want to have the freedom to explore, compare, analyze, and experiment.

Although these needs of the learner are quite obvious and readily endorsed by educators, there is developing an interesting turn of events, also related to efficiency and cost effectiveness, which on the surface, however, can appear to negate what is proposed above. To keep costs within reasonable limits for the learner, budgetary cuts in colleges and universities are sometimes resulting in reductions in the numbers of faculty positions while at the same time maintaining or even increasing numbers of students. One way for schools and departments of nursing to respond is by increasing the ratio of students to faculty. The phenomena is interesting in that, for years, nurse educators have equated low student–faculty ratios with higher quality education. But this is not necessarily the case. There is nothing magical about 1:5 or 1:7 or even 1:10 ratios.

Student–faculty ratios can be increased without decreasing the quality of education or safety to the client. What is needed to accomplish this is a rethinking of the purpose of the use of a laboratory and the teaching strategies to be used in conjunction with it. And, strangely enough, with high ratios and more independence of learning, the student may, in fact, be able to accomplish more effectively the program objectives related to professional judgment, critical thinking, creativity, and problem solving. To accomplish such objectives, the faculty member provides guidance instead of elbow supervision. The student learns not by having the faculty member at his elbow to direct him, but by having the faculty member guide him to the appropriate selection of problem-solving tasks that lead to an independent approach to testing theories.

In fact, the teacher does not need to be present at all times in the clinical setting. Careful teaching and planning for laboratory activities is of greater importance than the perpetual presence of the teacher.

A recent study produced some unexpected findings that tend to support this thesis.[2] Zanecchia's study, "A study of the relationships of nursing faculty attributes, faculty productivity, nursing student attributes and selected student outcomes," correlated a number of variables such as faculty–student ratios, tenure, doctoral status, number of publications, and years of teaching experience among others, with the pass rate on state board examinations. Surprisingly, a finding was that the smaller the number of faculty in a given program and the larger the ratios, the higher the pass rate on state board examinations. Could it be that faced with higher ratios these faculty found creative ways to deal with the numbers of students? And could it be that with more freedom and independence, these students functioned more effectively? Many questions arise and further study is needed, but the suggestion is there . . . if managed properly, higher faculty–student ratios have the potential for more effective learning.

Another study on new graduates found that there was no significant correlation between amount of clinical experience and test scores computed on study data in regard to associate degree and baccalaureate graduates.[3] Most of the correlations were on the negative side. So many questions arise in relation to the amount of time spent in clinical laboratory, although less time is *not* being advocated. Of late, there is concern for some programs using dangerously low numbers of hours in clinical laboratory. Perhaps the question is one of the use of the hours. All too often, time spent in clinical laboratory is used neither for learning what that setting has to offer or in giving service to clients. Too much time is spent "stumbling through the system" looking for equipment or discussing questions with the faculty member which at best suggests lack of prior learning for transfer to the situation at hand, mimicking performance of other nurses and/or the faculty member in order to comply with unstated expectations, or performing routine tasks. Cantor, et al.[3] concur when they state that:

> . . . nurse educators tend to plan the practicum around the existing hospital system, rather than using the hospital as a laboratory within which students learn about patients. Apparantly, nursing educators have not moved as far away from the approach of the past as they seem to believe. The major difference between nursing education today and the earlier programs seem to be shortened exposure to patient care experiences.

Obviously, the effectiveness of achieving desired outcomes and the efficiency of so doing are very much related in clinical teaching. The learners need to have assurance that their labs are likely to change their behavior in the desired direction and that their time and money is wisely used in the process. The most efficient use of the clinical laboratory, the optimal arrangement of activities within the laboratory, the most appropriate selection of settings, and the most efficient use of time within that setting is ultimately believed to contribute to effective learning.

Beyond effectiveness and efficiency, learners need to be provided with a challenge to learn that excites them and motivates them to progress in the program. Learning opportunities need to be varied, interesting, and different. Experimentation and successful problem solving provide an intrinsic reward system that propels the learner on to the next goal. The field of nursing needs more than even before to attract the best minds possible and to retain them. Nursing holds some of the most exciting challenges available among career choices. Learners need to be led to unlock those challenges and partake in them. There is much to offer career-minded men and women; the secret is for the educator to convey this and for the learner to discover it.

The learner in nursing education, like other students, is more sophisticated than ever before. Expectations are understandably high. They are a part of a heterogeneous group of students, from various backgrounds, a wide age span, and with a broad spectrum of personal responsibilities and goals. Many fall into the category of adult learners. They expect an approach to learning that takes these factors into account. For example, they want to play an active role in goal achievement; they are accustomed to making decisions for themselves, and they have learned to be creative problem solvers. The learner-centered elements not only meet the needs of the immediate post-high school student, but are most appropriate for the adult learner. When used to their fullest extent, they have the potential for greatly satisfying the needs of all learners, and for producing a competent graduate.

Facilitation of Learning by the Faculty

In short, to facilitate desired learning and maintain optimal student interest in clinical laboratory activities, the teaching strategies of nurse faculty should be geared to stimulate thinking, challenge what has already been learned, and facilitate what the student would like to learn. The faculty member must behave very much like a teacher and not as a nurse.

Guidance rather than elbow supervision is required; raising questions rather than answering them; providing cues rather than prescriptive assignments; "setting the stage" rather than "acting out the performance." Of course, the focus must always be on learning rather than caring, except at the end of the program of study when students are ready to integrate all learnings and test their application to caring as a whole. And, to do this a wide range of agency and nonagency clinical settings are required. The faculty member must know them well to guide students through them efficiently and effectively.

Novel approaches to assignment of students to clinical facilities could be tested. Opportunity to have a wide exposure to acute care, health promotion, and long-term care facilities need to be used. Yet, expecting students to merely move from one type of agency to another, and even to community resources such as schools that are not specifically geared to health care, can result in a number of fragmented activities without a unifying theme. Rather than structuring the traditional rotations, other arrangements utilizing segments of the community as a whole could be tried.

For example, a regional approach to assignments is useful. A team of faculty representing areas of specialization in nursing is assigned to a geographic region consisting perhaps of an urban and suburban area. The region has certain characteristic features that impact on health, such as industrial blue collar, or high technology, business, white collar workers. Then the hospitals, ambulatory care services, mental health centers, home health care services, schools, and so forth are used for student practice. The group of students assigned to the team of faculty would move about within the region for a term or semester to fulfill clinical objectives. More freedom is thereby afforded both faculty and students, a broader view of nursing is developed, and the client is afforded more continuity of care. Other patterns of assignment might be designed to afford similar goal achievement.

**Consideration of the Client/Consumer
in the Clinical Laboratory**

The basic right and expectations of clients are to quality care. Conversely, then, quality care is not a privilege reserved for a few, or received under some circumstances and not under others. Therefore, quality care can be expected by all clients from all practitioners of nursing. The quality service in any field is expected from its practicing professionals. The responsibility for delivering, guiding, and overseeing such service is invested in these professionals.

In educational programs for the professions, such as nursing, segments of client care are entrusted to students for periods of time for purposes of learning. At least two issues arise in relation to the client who is the consumer of nursing care. The first is that of the quality of the care; secondly, there is the issue of assuring the privacy of the client. While it is difficult enough to assure both of these elements in nursing care rendered by expert practitioners, it indeed becomes increasingly difficult to protect the privacy of people and control for quality when nursing students are introduced in a wide variety of settings. Yet, the intents are not impossible to fulfill.

First, as far as quality care is concerned, the best insurance for that is a knowledgeable and skillful care-giver. Knowledge and skill are requisite whether the care-giver is a licensed practitioner or a student. So, it would follow that a less than knowledgeable student has the potential for subjecting a client to a lower quality of care, questionable safety levels, and even to the risk of increased costs.

Under the use of the clinical laboratory being proposed in this book, a knowledgeable, skillful learner is provided in each clinical situation. Each skill objective presupposes acquisition of tested knowledge, demonstration of skill in the college laboratory, and readiness for transfer of learning to the real situation. The student is responsible for and accountable to others for his/her own actions. Throughout the process being proposed, the student must display a level of knowledge and skill prerequisite to clinical activities. The result is expected to be a higher quality of interaction with the client as well as a higher margin of safety to the client. And, as far as safety is concerned, the proposed use of the college laboratory provides a measure of competency before the student encounters clients in the clinical laboratory. So, faculty provide for safety of clients through what the student knows and not through what the teacher does.

As far as the privacy of the client is concerned, this area presents a set of problems that are more difficult to handle. And there are no clear-cut solutions. For, as students move away from rendering "total care" to clients, and move into accomplishing objectives directed at learning the component parts of caring, more students are observing more clients, asking more questions, and taking up more time of clients and even the practitioners. In many instances, each client would have contact with increased numbers of students. For example, three students may present to a client in the course of a day to make certain observations; in the traditional model of assignments, one student would spend a concentrated period with this client and make the observations while giving care.

Most importantly, practitioners and educators alike must respect the right of clients to decline in participation of activites with students. Free choice must be offered. If clients permit students to participate in their care, then the intrusions into their rest and privacy should be within reason and the ultimate respect for the person. Yet, nursing students might be afforded no more, but no less than other health professional students. Medical students, for instance, move about a general hospital, in and out of clients rooms, to take histories, listen to heart sounds, make observations, etc. So, this pattern of assignment for learning is not without precedent. Nurse educators and nursing students need to rethink the process of learning and the needs of clients in order to balance the desires of both.

At least one distinct advantage to the consumer in this system is that because care is entrusted to an expert practitioner and students participate in aspects of care, the costs to the client for service are actually attributed to the service by nursing service personnel. Conversely, students are shouldering only the costs of learning and are not contributing to service.

It is not clear that we have paid enough attention to the problems surrounding the client in settings in which health professional education is provided. Much more exploration is needed. By and large, in a society growing in affluence, the client wishes to be an active participant in decisions affecting care.

Cooperation and Support of Educational Administrators, Nursing Service Personnel, and Agency Administrators

The administrators of educational programs and health care agencies, as well as the practitioners of nursing in nursing service, all play a vital role in the process of clinical teaching. Yet the roles are not always clear and optimal outcomes are not always achieved. Their roles, together with the nurse educator role are complementary.

The major role of the administrator of the educational unit is twofold: to facilitate the student placements selected by the faculty and to contract for the needed educational activities with the agencies involved. Educational administrators need to place the responsibility for selecting clinical settings on the faculty. Faculty are in the best position to determine which settings will facilitate the accomplishment of objectives. Also, faculty carry the responsibility for the initial contacts with appropriate agency personnel to explore the possibilities of an agreement. In this phase, the educational adminstrator is an important facilitator in terms of enhancing contacts with agency personnel, contributing on an informal basis to positive interpersonal relationships, and to maintaining a positive image of the educational institution in the community.

When an understanding is reached between the faculty members involved and the agency personnel as to the use of the agency's facilities by students, then the formal contract is signed by the administrators of the educational institution and service agency. As the use of clinical laboratory in nursing education evolves along different lines, contract language needs to be adjusted to reflect the intent of the agreement. For example, in the conceptualization of the use of the clinical laboratory by Glass,[4] she speaks of a "fluidity of movement" of students and faculty in settings. As expectations regarding student activities change, both parties need to provide for such understandings in contract language. The educational administrator plays a leadership role in the design and implementation of the contract.

The role of the agency administrators is to hear the needs to nursing education and to cooperate wherever possible to match these needs with available resources in their agencies. Atraditional requests on behalf of students may seem burdensome initially, but providing a testing ground for new teaching strategies in their settings would be extremely helpful. Such an "investment" on their part today could yield more competent practitioners tomorrow. Retaining traditional educational practices only reinforces the status quo.

Staff nurses need to be very much involved in communicating with nurse faculty in the potential uses of their units for student learning. Ultimately, it is the staff nurses who are the most involved and most valuable resources to the students. Their input into planning and decision making is of the utmost importance. Some of these practitioners may serve as preceptors. This role is discussed more fully in the next chapter. These nurses are to be aware of the educational needs and fully cognizant of their important contribution to the learning of students.

Some scrutiny of the long-standing relationship between educational and health service institutions reveals, in many instances, a rather one-sided or parasitic relationship. Educators have been the takers, consistently on the receiving end of the relationship. The expectation has been that agencies will afford their clients, space, practitioners, and other resources to faculty and students with limited tangible returns in exchange. Actually, it is true that the most valuable return to them should be quality graduates who will become their practitioners.

Nevertheless, in return for the cooperation gained from both agency and nonagency personnel, faculty need to assume responsibility for determining what can be offered to these people in return for what is expected from them. For example, regular annual of semiannual meetings with them would be aimed at helping them understand the curriculum, the objectives, and their role in accomplishing them. Also, a clear articulation of changing faculty roles is essential because they are likely to conflict with traditional expectations. Large group meetings afford the opportunity for service personnel to share perspectives and suggestions, as well as socialize with their colleagues. If these meetings are held on the campus, there is the added advantage of offering the opportunity to practicing nurses to become reacquainted with the atmosphere of academia. Additionally, in such meetings nurse faculty are challenged to articulate their role and their program—and they must believe in it if they are to articulate it and convince others of its worth.

Additionally, educators can offer service agencies consultation by faculty, as well as inservice or continuing education workshops conducted by faculty. Such endeavors would have cyclic benefits to all involved. Faculty would have influence on upgrading the level of practice in settings used by students; in turn, the staff nurses could serve as desirable role models for the students. Faculty could help to develop the use of conceptual models and care plans by nurses; student learning would be facilitated in the "real world", and faculty would have more desirable circumstances in which to conduct their own research and practice. Also, faculty assistance in guiding staff nurses to identify research problems and design research protocols would be much appreciated. These and other faculty gestures that demonstrate interest in nursing service and an appreciation for their cooperation could only help to improve that much needed relationship. We need each other.

To facilitate communication between and among the personnel involved in clinical activities, faculty would do well to share curricular goals and materials in writing as well as verbally. The description of the school's philosophy, program objectives, conceptual framework, and course syllabi could be distributed and discussed. In addition to these items, a different approach to clinical teaching such as has been described, may be more acceptable to agency personnel if it were to be clearly articulated in writing.

For example, a statement of philosophy of the school's use of the college laboratory and clinical laboratory would convey values that could serve as the basis for discussion and testing. It would also serve to clarify inter- and intrafaculty views. Included in such statements may be the following.

> The college laboratory serves as an initial step in the application of knowledge to care and in the application of theory to practice.
>
> Use of the college laboratory is believed to broaden a student's comprehension of selected aspects of problems of the real world that may not be available to each student within the clinical laboratory. It thereby provides a predictable means for achieving course objectives and serves as a logical progression to the real-life situation of the clinical laboratory.
>
> Clinical laboratory provides opportunity for client contact. Client contact is essential for learning to care, and it is utilized when it furnishes the best means of goal achievement, that is, when a goal cannot be accomplished in the classroom or college laboratory. Contacts with clients are designed to allow students to learn to apply knowledge to care of clients. Early in the program of study students learn to apply knowledge to selected aspects of care; later in the program of clinical study students learn to give comprehensive care to clients."[5]

More concrete statements of responsibility of faculty, students, and agency personnel could then follow. These statements or guidelines provide a clearer view of how each person proceeds in the clinical laboratory based on the philosophical stance put forth. For example,

The faculty member:
> Determines with the student the need for, or lack of need for, the presence of the faculty member in the clinical laboratory setting.
>
> Structures clinical laboratory activities so that the student experiments with and discovers new insights into problems of client care.
>
> Serves as a consultant to agencies in one's area of expertise.

The student:
> Participates in the selection of clinical laboratory activities.
>
> Communicates with agency personnel regarding activities within that agency.
>
> Accepts responsibility to prepare for competent, safe practice in the clinical laboratory and to seek faculty validation of achievement.

The agency personnel:
> Retain accountability for the quality of client care; students retain accountability for their own actions.

Serve as valuable resource persons to students, but are not expected to assume the role of teacher. Students who appear to lack knowledge or skill related to the activities engaged in should be referred to the faculty member.[6]

Nurse educators need quality care settings to use for clinical practice; nursing service personnel need quality products in the form of graduates to staff their facilities. Nurse educators carry the weighty responsibility of blending the immediate and long-term needs of both to produce a harmonious, productive relationship. Administrators in the academic setting need to free faculty to select clinical activities in a variety of settings. Administrators in service institutions need to permit practicing nurses the time and opportunity to work with nursing faculty and students.

At the same time there needs to be a clear understanding and commitment to the goals of the teaching institution by the administrators and practitioners of service agencies. Faculty have the responsibility to clearly articulate expected roles and relationships and to convince service personnel of their value.

For practitioners, the clinical setting is a place to render service; for educators, it's a place to facilitate student learning. The so-called confusion between "service" and "education" can be dispelled by clearly articulating and depicting relationships, establishing open and consistent communication channels, and mutually recognizing and respecting the contributions of each to quality nursing care. Practitioners need to be utilized as active partners in the educational process with something to gain as well as something to contribute. Nurse faculty have the responsibility to serve as consultants, liaison persons, and resources for continuing education in settings that cooperate with educational institutions. Nurse faculty also have the responsibility to involve staff in research projects.

Such cooperative activities are expected to upgrade the level of practice and shape the role model of the nurse for students in the settings.

Notes

1. Reilly, D. *Perspectives on the clinical laboratory in baccalaureate nursing education: Developing compentency and maximizing resources,* Unpublished paper presented at an invitational conference for educators in baccalaureate nursing education, Paper II, Medical College of Ohio, Toledo, Ohio, March 30, 1983.
2. Zanecchia, M. D. *A study of the relationships of nursing faculty attributes, faculty productivity, nursing student attributes and selected*

student outcomes. Unpublished doctoral dissertation, Storrs, Connecticut, University of Connecticut, 1981.

3. Cantor, M. M, Schroeder, D. M., & Kurth, S. W. The experienced nurse and the new graduate: Do their learning needs differ? *Nurse Educator,* 1981,6 (7), 17–22.

4. Glass, H. P. *Teaching behavior in the nursing laboratory in selected baccalaureate nursing programs in Canada.* Unpublished doctoral dissertation, New York, Teachers College, Columbia University, 1971.

5. Excerpts from the "Philosophy of Laboratory" of the University of Connecticut School of Nursing.

6. Excerpts from the "Guidelines for Use of the Clinical Laboratory" of the University of Connecticut School of Nursing.

Bibliography

Cantor, M. M., Schroeder, D. M., Kurth, S. W. The experienced nurse and the new graduate: Do their learning needs differ? *Nurse Educator,* 1981, 6 (7), 17–22.

Durrant, L. The student of nursing needs—The consumer of education. *Journal of Nursing Education,* 1978, 78 (6), 15–19.

Fischback, F. M. Personal growth and learning of students in an open-ended clinical experience: A motivational philosophy. *Journal of Nursing Education,* 1977, 16 (2), 30–33.

Hemelt, M. D., & Mackert, M. E. *Dynamics of law in nursing and health care.* Reston, Virginia: Reston Publishers, 1982.

Lazinski, H. The effect of clinical teaching on the budgets of schools of nursing. *Journal of Nursing Education,* 1979, 18 (1), 21–24.

Samples, B. *The metaphoric mind.* Reading, Massachusetts: Addison-Wesley Publishing Company, 1976.

Tetreault, A. I. Selected factors associated with professional attitude of baccalaureate nursing students. *Nursing Research,* 1976, 25 (1), 49–53.

Treece, E. M. Students' opinions concerning patient selection for clinical practice. *Journal of Nursing Education,* 1969, 8 (2), 17–21, 24–25.

CHAPTER 7

Use of Preceptors in the Clinical Laboratory

As the field of nursing began to mature into a profession, the need to prepare its new practitioners in the art and science of nursing was well recognized. It became readily apparent that on-the-job training would not suffice. To delineate the "before the fact" preparation of its practitioners from the "after the fact" practice by its practitioners, a number of revolutionary changes began to occur. In essence, nursing education distinguished itself from nursing service; nurse educators held positions apart from head nurses and nursing service personnel; nursing students became distinguishable from nurses by their activities; learning, at least to some extent, has been distinguished from practice. Nursing education even "changed its address" to facilitate this change; it moved to the college campus, away from the hospital settings devoted to practice.

Whereas all of these distinctions were imperative and much has been gained by nursing in this long and difficult process, the two worlds of nursing education and nursing practice grew further apart. And by necessity it needed to be so: first, to clearly identify the different missions of the two, and secondly to funnel the paucity of well-prepared nurses into positions in nursing education. Those with degrees were expected to teach. And the struggle to staff our schools and departments with faculty who possess credentials equal to their counterparts in other schools and departments on the campus continues. So, the route that was taken to achieve the goal was a reasonable one. However, the problems that ensued were developmental in nature, and to be expected, but nursing education and nursing service grew farther apart. They even became competitive; as if they were working toard separate goals. In actuality the goal of both is quality nursing care. And the structure, activities, and function of each could and should be complementary.

Nursing currently is in a position to more fully recognize the complementary roles of nursing education and nursing service. There is a readiness for this. Nurse educators are more secure: They are achieving doctorates in greater numbers, and even those with masters degrees are involved in scholarly activities. Curricula are quite respectable and are utilizing theory to guide practice. In nursing practice, more nurses have earned or are earning graduate education than ever before. There is more of a curiosity about ways to contribute to quality practice. They are ripe for modeling good practice to students and having more influcence on the thinking and actions of nursing students.

At the same time, nurse educators have matured to the point where they envision possibilities and even advantages to having practitioners participate in the educational process. Oddly enough, this realization is dawning at a time when budgetary demands in educational institutions coupled with evoling faculty role issues, such as faculty practice time, are forcing nurse faculty to find ways to use their own time more effectively and efficiently. Such considerations would also free them for research and writing activities.

It is understandable that nurse faculty moved through a period in which they expected to be all things to all students. Only recently are they realizing that educators alone cannot accomplish this in a professional field. But faculty, when socialized into the role of nurse, were instructed to think this way—nurses were led to believe that they should be all things to their "patients." And they were led to believe that they could satisfy all needs and give total care; as if that were possible. As faculty then, there is a need to retrain modes of thinking to be facilitators, influence others, and capitalize on resource people. In fact, by so doing, the learning of students might be broadened and enhanced.

One way to accomplish that is to utilize clinical preceptors in clinical settings to provide some clinical guidance of nursing students.[1] Besides providing a potential solution to some practical problems, a clinical preceptor model(s) could actually strengthen the ties between nursing service and nursing education. Although there has been limited use of preceptorships in nursing education, its use has been largely in relation to the clinical practice of graduate students. Its value in graduate education is generally appreciated, but the concept could be extended into undergraduate preparation for nurses.

What follows is a limited discussion of the use of clinical preceptors in nursing education. This brief treatise is intended to attest to the growing importance of preceptorships in clinical teaching and to provide some basic

guidelines for nurse educators. Fuller discussions on the subject of preceptorships are emerging.[2] In the literature, words are used in a similar manner, but may convey somewhat different meanings. Hence, the following set
of definitions.

PRECEPTOR. One who guides, tutors, provides direction aimed at a specific performance.

ROLE MODEL. One who demonstrates desired behaviors and values.

MENTOR. A wise and trusted counselor. A seasoned professional who
counsels the novice in the use of knowledge, skills, and attitudes in a given
field.

RESOURCE. One who serves as an available support and aid through his or
her intellectual or personal capabilities.

A clinical preceptor is expected to depict the seasoned practitioner of
nursing and serve as a resource person to the student. The clinical preceptor is
not expected to teach or to replace any of the guidance activities of the
teacher discussed in the preceding chapters. In other words, use of a clinical
preceptor is not intended to replace the nurse faculty member, but rather to
complement the role of the faculty person in the clinical laboratory. The

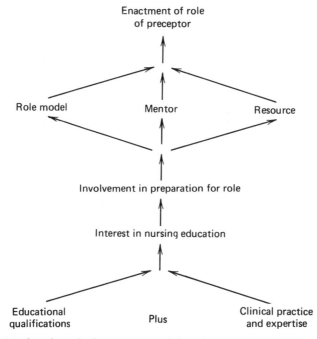

Figure 7.1 Flow chart of role components of clinical preceptors in nursing education.

clinical preceptor is familiar with the academic program, the course objectives and activities, and can guide the student to appropriate clients, health team members, and facilities to fulfill objectives.

The preceptor role is conceptualized as embodying that of role model, mentor, and resource person. Figure 7.1 depicts the various facets of qualifications, preparation, and enactment of the role of clinical preceptor.

Selection of Appropriate Preceptors

Not every nurse could or should be a clinical preceptor to nursing students. A combination of special personal and professional qualities are desirable. Even the resulting combination needs to be special. The nurse needs to exude an enthusiasm for nursing practice that is contagious. This person must be someone who is very successful in their position. Helmuth and Guberski[3] summarize this person well:"The nurse planning to be a preceptor needs a strong educational and experiential background, a special program of study, and the opportunity to work with an experienced preceptor." The faculty member needs to be cognizant of such qualifications to make selections that have the potential for advantageous outcomes.

Educational qualifications are an important determinant. The clinical preceptor ideally holds at least one academic degree beyond that being earned by the student. So for the graduate students the norm would be the doctorate and for the undergraduates the norm would be the masters degree. Because the world of practice does not afford the numbers of nurses with this educational preparation, the masters degree more often is found to be the norm. Most schools aspire to clinical preceptors holding the same minimal educational qualifications as their faculty, and that is the masters degree. In addition, the other basic qualification is that the preceptor must be clinically expert. This nurse must be a master practitioner who continues to practice and work on improving practice. Various measures could be used to determine this level of expertise; foremost among them is certification in one of the practice areas by the American Nurses' Assocation (ANA). Some other measures may be specialty related, regional, or even institutionally derived. At any rate, clinical preceptors should have something special to offer in their practice.

Additionally, a potential preceptor should be highly respected by nurse colleagues and other health professionals. The extent of this reputation should be at least throughout the employing institution, but preferably on a regional basis. Recognized leadership qualities by health team members attest to this reputation. Often, this area of achievement is derived through seeking appropriate consultation on a regional or even national basis, and participating in collaborative interactions from the most narrow to the broadest sense, that is, from regular health team conferences on a nursing unit, to regional planning conferences and health association programs. Visibility provides a means of continuing evaluation and credibility.

Preceptor participation in clinical research on an ongoing basis is growing in importance as undergraduate and graduate students alike use the research process as the very basis for their nursing actions. Serving as an investigator, coinvestigator, or staff member on a research probject is illustrative to students of the role they are expected to assume. Involving students in even small ways with such on going projects provides the finest stimulus for their own conduct of clinical research. Also, the practitioner who is involved in research is more likely to portray further desirable characteristics involving a curiosity to learn and a flexible approach to learning and practicing nursing. This nurse is likely to be more concerned with testing approaches to practice as opposed to conveying facts, figures, and a specific way to perform skills simply because "we've always done it this way." In fact, a clinical preceptor should welcome probing questions, some of which have no answers currently, and be able to deal successfully with a level of uncertainity.

Students need to view a practicing nurse who is confident, independent, assertive, and self-assured. Faculty and students would not pose a threat, but rather a challenge to this type of person. And think of the challenge such a person would pose to the student in regard to role taking. Furthermore, the preceptor should be able to inspire and support the student in the clinical area while fostering independence of action as an end product. The entire purpose of precepting would be defeated if the student became dependent on the preceptor. This is no more desirable than the student becoming dependent on the faculty member.

Finally, faculty need to select potential preceptors who are very much involved in the actual practice of nursing. This is very important for faculty to explore because so many graduate prepared nurses are heavily invested in management functions. Such a nurse is, of course, a good preceptor for a graduate student in a management course, but not for an undergraduate or graduate student in a clinical course focused on the care of clients. Together with a heavy practice role, this nurse must be interested in participating in the educational process. Not all nurses who meet the above characteristics are interested in cooperating with an educational program. Hopefully, such an interest will grow among practitioners of nursing as a part of accountability for the future of the profession of nursing.

Faculty Preparation of Preceptors

Even the most eligible candidates cannot be expected to succeed as clinical preceptors for students without an orderly system of preparation for the role. Faculty members carry the responsibility for conducting initial as well as ongoing preparation of the preceptor for the role. Such a system could be implemented formally or informally, individually or in groups. The following points to be included in such a system are not intended to be exhaustive, but rather exemplary of the type of attention needed in an orientation process.

1. Possession of and articulation of the course syllabus.
2. Provision of a detailed letter of agreement written by the faculty member.
3. Approval from the administrators under whom the nurse functions for participation in this role.
4. Clear delineation of the characteristics, functions, and responsibilities of the clinical preceptor. It may also be desirable to generate a set of guidelines or behaviors for proceeding in the role.
5. Clear delineation of faculty role in the teaching–learning process. Note the complementary roles of the teacher and preceptor. Include a clear identification of the student objectives and clinical activities.
6. Removal of responsibilities of teaching and evaluation from the preceptor. These responsibilities are inherent in the faculty role. Sharing the evaluation tools can be useful. The preceptor could utilize such tools to collect and systematically share useful data with the faculty member.
7. Allowance of time for both formal and informal feedback by the preceptor to the faculty member. The process involves the reverse as well.
8. Facilitation of on going administrative support in the clinical setting.
9. Provision of the personal and professional support that assist the preceptor to cope with expected role conflict. Relief of guilt and means to optimal functioning in dual roles is often the object of such support, as the preceptor attempts to divide both time and attention between the student and the demands of the practice role.
10. Determination of an acceptable reward system involving professional exchange rather than monetary rewards. Sustain interest in and desirability for the role without incurring financial constraints. In some instances clinical faculty appointments for preceptors are appropriate. The system should be based on perceived mutual benefits.
11. Development of an ongoing evaluation method for the overall process by the faculty member. This would serve as a means of improving the relationship over time.

Such a working arrangement has much potential for an enriching experience among faculty, students, and practicing nurses. Acceptable reward systems for preceptors need to be continually evaluated.

Role of Preceptors

The role of the clinical preceptor as suggested here involves three facets: role model, mentor, and resource person.

Role Model. Role models teach by their actions. They model desirable behaviors of nursing practice such as making valid professional judgments and using the norms of critical thinking. Tobiason[4] so aptly describes role modeling as a learning process that involves identification and internalization. The learner observes the model's behavior and eventually internalizes the values on which that behavior is based.

Clinical preceptors model behaviors that are planned for observation by students, however, many valuable behaviors are chance happenings. Hence, a long-term relationship between the student and preceptor provides additional benefits. In essence, the role model shows a student how to proceed in the real world. The student is thereby assisted to acquire an identity as a nurse. Role socialization is facilitated.

Mentor. The clinical preceptor serves as a mentor rather than a teacher to the student. One role enhances the other. Specific mentor actions include suggesting client-related activities appropriate to the knowledge base and skill level of the learner. Discussion of such activities within the context of the program's conceptual framework would follow. Mentors observe aspects of student–client interaction, react to data collected, critique health assessments, validate findings, and critique proposed management plans. Throughout this relationship the student is queried and prodded into independent decision making and is assisted in self-evaluation. The mentor leads a student to a higher level of functioning in clinical settings without being directive.

Resource Person. The clinical preceptor knows the agency or institution and its personnel better than the faculty member. To facilitate the use of clinical time for learning and to avoid wasting time "stumbling through the the system," the resource person role becomes very valuable. Students should be introduced to health professionals involved in the care of clients. They should be informed of who is conducting health-related research projects. The resource person also acquaints students with the variety of services and support programs that could relate to student assignments. Again, providing cues, introducing key persons, and making subtle suggestions are desired rather than providing direction or structured use of available resources.

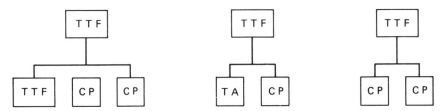

Figure 7.2 Use of preceptors in clinical teaching. TTF, tenure tract faculty; CP, clinical preceptor; TA, teaching assistant.

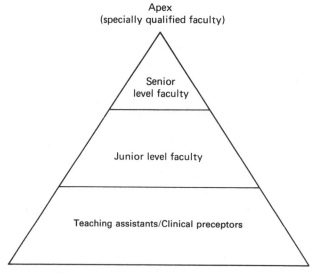

Figure 7.3 Pyramid model of clinical teaching.

A variety of models for the use of clinical preceptors could be tested (Figures 7.2 and 7.3). These models propose a use of clinical preceptors and include the use of teaching assistants. While teaching assistants (TAs) are often used for tasks not involving student interactions, that is, test item analyses, administering tests, grading, ordering books, and preparing handouts and media, some TAs could assume some responsibility for clinical teaching. Doctoral candidates who are TAs could participate in clinical activities with both undergraduate and graduate students of nursing.

The pyramid model of teaching consists of a team of one expert teacher with lesser prepared team members. This model permits a senior faculty member or a tenure tract faculty member to have larger sections of students with assistance in clinical activities from junior faculty, TAs, and clinical preceptors.

Such an expanded view of clinical teaching in nursing education could not only serve to enhance the teaching–learning process, but results in a closer, collaborative relationship between nursing education and nursing service. More joint research projects involving educators and practitioners are likely to result. They are novel to nursing education. But other disciplines have used a combination of these strategies with a fair amount of success.

The problem of dealing with the financial responsibilities of education and service remain and need to be studied. No single plan or system would be appropriate to every school or agency. Models need to be tested. Yet the proposed working relationship seems to hold promise for the future.

Notes

1. Helmuth, M. R., & Guberski, T. D. Preparation for preceptor role. *Nursing Outlook*, 1980, *28* (1), 36–39.
2. Stuart-Siddall, S., & Haberlin, J. M. *Preceptorships in nursing education.* Rockville, Maryland: Aspent Systems Corporation, 1983.
3. Op cit., Helmuth, M. R., & Guberski, T. D., 36–39.
4. Tobiason, S. J. A plea to role models. *Supervisor Nurse*, 1979, *10* (1), 36–37.

Bibliography

Atwood, A. R. The mentor in clinical practice. *Nursing Outlook*, 1979, *27* (11), 714–717.

Blazeck, A. M., Selekman, J., Timpe, M., & Wolf, E. R. Unification: Nursing education and nursing practice. *Nursing and Health Care*, 1982, *3* (1), 18–24.

Chickerella, B. G., & Lutz, W. J. Professional nurturance: Preceptorships for undergraduate nursing students. *American Journal of Nursing*, 1981, *81* (1), 107–109.

Dienemann, J. Reducing nursing faculty workloads without increasing costs. *Image: The Journal of Nursing Scholarship*, 1983, *15* (4), 111–114.

Friesen, L., & Conahan, B. J. A clinical preceptor program: Strategy for new graduate orientation. *Journal of Nursing Administration*, 1980, *10* (4), 18–23.

Helmuth, M. R., & Guberski, T. D. Preparation for preceptor role. *Nursing Outlook*, 1980, *28* (1), 36–39.

Kelly, L. Y. Power guide—The mentor relationship. *Nursing Outlook*, 1978, *26* (5), 339.

Limon, S., Bargagliotti, A., & Spencer, J. B. Who precepts the preceptor? *Nursing and Health Care*, 1981, *2* (8), 433–436.

Morton, P. G. The financial distress of higher education: Impact on nursing. *Image: The Journal of Nursing Scholarship*, 1983, *15* (4), 102–106.

Murphy, M. L., Hammerstand, S. M. Preparing a staff nurse for precepting. *Nurse Educator*, 1981, *6* (5), 17–20.

Pardue, S. F. The who-what-why of mentor teacher/graduate student relationships. *Journal of Nursing Education*, 1983, *22* (1), 32–37.

Sherman, J. E. Role modeling for FNP students. *Nursing Outlook*, 1980, *23* (1), 40–42.

Simon, J. L. *A role guide and resource book for clinical preceptors.* U.S. Department of HEW, Publication No. (HRA) 7–14.

Stuart-Siddal, S., & Haberlin, J. M. *Preceptorships in nursing education.* Rockville, Maryland: Aspen Systems Corporation, 1983.

Walters, C. R. Using staff preceptors in a senior experience. *Nursing Outlook*, 1981, *29* (4), 245–247.

Westcot, L. B. Nursing education and nursing service: A collaborative model. *Nursing and Health Care*, 1981, *21* (7), 376–379.

CHAPTER 8

Use of Evaluation Methods to Determine Achievement in Clinical Practice

Most nurse educators would agree with Irby and Dohner[1] who comment that "Evaluation of student clinical performance is one of the most complex areas of the teaching/learning process in the health professions." The study of clinical evaluation has been much discussed and described. Obviously, there are no easy or clear-cut answers to the questions posed by educators. Yet, the subject is of such great importance to a practice field like nursing that the struggle to improve performance testing and grading continues. Actually, as is the case with all aspects of evaluation, the aim of the evaluator is to objectify, to whatever extent possible, a heavily value laden or subjective process. Educators in all fields know that this is difficult enough to accomplish in the cognitive realm and paper and pencil testing, but, the difficulties are both magnified and multiplied in practice fields where performance testing, that is, in the psychomotor realm, is a critical component of the teacher's judgment as to the progression and graduation of students. All teaching and evaluation in a professional or practice field is aimed at the rendering of a quality service. Also, some aspects of the affective domain are evaluated in clinical practice.

The previous discussion of teaching strategies recommended in both the college laboratory and the clinical laboratory has implications for clinical evaluation. In fact, changing views of the use of clinical laboratory for teach-

148

ing and learning produce interesting dilemmas for the evaluation of the learner in that setting. Some traditional views regarding evaluation of student performance require scrutiny and adjustment, particularly in relation to what is evaluated, when, and how. The nurse educator searches for evaluation methods that are appropriate to psychomotor skill achievement and attitudinal development. The evaluator begins to appreciate that the entire process must support the degree of freedom and creativity that was fostered in the learner throughout the teaching–learning process. Evaluation methods with such characteristics are not easy to come by.

Additionally, the teaching needs to be continually cognizant of the notion that evaluation and grading are two separate processes. Evaluation may lead to grading, but separate considerations need to be made of each. And there should be congruency between the methods selected for evaluation and grading. Although this chapter is not intended to present a comprehensive discussion of the subject of evaluation or grading, a brief review of the concepts underlying each will be presented. Consultation of major sources in this area is assumed.

Evaluation

Evaluation involves the judging of the worth or effectiveness of an experience or process. In nursing education a series of activities leading to student experiences are planned and guided to produce a nurse. Hence, evaluation is extremely important to judging the worth or effectiveness of those activities through the demonstrated behaviors of the student. Being a health service oriented profession, evaluation in nursing education is also important to preserve the safety of the public to be served by that new practitioner.

The discussion of evaluation will be limited to that of student performance. Program evaluation is a separate part of education. The focus of the "judging" is in relation to measurable student behaviors. The students behaviors are those that are expected to flow from and be in concert with stated behavioral objectives.

The word *evaluation* embodies the word *value*. The value system of the evaluator is inadvertently contained in the methods selected and the processes instituted to make the judgments. So by its very nature, the evaluation process is heavily laden with subjectivity. As mentioned earlier, the task of the evaluator is to control for subjectivity as much as possible. In the following discussion it can be noted that the "value of the educator toward the process of evaluation" can be used to advantage. Basically, subjectivity in judgments should be controlled for, but the evaluator's values for what, when, and how evaluation should occur can be shaped on the basis of knowledge of evaluation in skill performance and in consideration of the needs to the learner. The latter point is aimed at avoiding placing the person to be evaluated at a disadvantage, so that the judgments are unfair and invalid.

One way to avoid this problem is to understand that evaluation is not an end in itself. Instead, evaluation is a process intended to achieve an end—specifically stated learnings translated into behaviors. The process is intended to be positive and productive. So the behavioral objectives are the end point, and the evaluation process is a means to achieve that end.

Secondly, the evaluation process has been described as having two phases.[2] These two phases are formative evaluation and summative evaluation. Although the model developed by Scriven[2] was for program evaluation, it is presently applied to student performance. Formative evaluation of performance provides teacher feedback of the progression being made by the learner toward goal achievement. The teacher molds the learner in the shape of desired behaviors. Formative evaluation should be nonjudgmental and provide hints and suggestions rather than negative criticism. Positive comments and reinforcements of desired behaviors are constructive. The teacher suggests cues to future action; the learner combines the cues with past learning to embark on new insights and higher quality practices. The aim of formative evaluation is guidance toward achievement of stated outcomes. Formative evaluation can be provided weekly through individual conferences and written comments.

On the other hand, summative evaluation of performance provides statements of the extent of achievement of objectives or goals. Summative evaluation conveys judgments made at a specified point in time, that is, the end of a semester. Summative evaluation presupposes that formative has been done at regular intervals throughout the allotted period of learning. The performances judged at that point are those in relation to the behavioral objectives. The aim of summative evaluation is a summation of outcome performances as displayed at a specific time.

Grading

Grading is a process separate from, and following upon, evaluation. It presents a unique set of problems and concerns. According to Dressel and Nelson,[3] "There is no solution to the grading problem satisfactory to all concerned. Students would like all As, administrators would like few Fs, and the teachers would like to be left alone." A commentary most experienced teachers would readily agree with.

But , of course, grading is demanded in most segments of higher education as a matter of educational policy and as a means to convey to society the level of academic achievement of individuals. So, grading needs to be done;

the system used and its meaning needs to be consistent and well understood by faculty and students alike. Yet, preoccupation with grading by either group can be detrimental to the teaching–learning process.

A grade is a symbol that represents a level of student achievement in a course of study. Generally, the grade is a letter and is summative in nature, that is, it is assigned at the end of the course of study. In grading clinical performance, the grade assigned by the teacher is usually substantiated by a narrative description of accomplishments.

A grade can be arrived at on the basis of normative referenced standards. Normative references standards are based on relative standards; one student is considered relative to another. The standard is the average performance of the group and each student's achievement is compared against the others in the class. A bell curve is assumed. So, for example, if in a group of 100 students, normative referenced standards are applied and A to F grading is in effect, approximately 10% of the students would be assigned an A, 20 to 25% would get a B, 30 to 40% would get a C, 20 to 25% would get a D, and approximately 10% would get an F.

Criterion referenced standards are based on predetermined, explicitly stated criteria. In performance testing, the criteria are stated in behavioral terms. Each student's performance is compared to the stated criteria, so that an absolute, as opposed to a relative standard, is used in interpreting the behaviors.

Considering each of the basic concepts briefly presented, the following discussion of clinical evaluation and grading demonstrates application of these concepts. Additionally, this discussion reflects the application of the essential elements of clinical teaching discussed in previous chapters. For example, the active involvement of the learner in clinical teaching is extended to clinical evaluation in which the active involvement of the learner is also advocated. An attempt is made to *suggest approaches* to the process of clinical evaluation; prescriptive methods are not presented. That aspect is left to individual faculties to design according to their philosophy, conceptual framework, arrangement of content, and academic calendar.

The following discussion is divided into four parts: standards, processes, tools, and measurements.

Standards

A standard is a principle, rule, model, or pattern against which to compare the quantity, excellence, or correctness of other patterns or performances. The standards for clinical evaluation to be considered are: clearly stated behaviors upon which to determine performance expectations, timing of the evaluation, sampling of performances, level of performance, and perceptions of the student regarding evaluation standards.

In clinical evaluation the standards are the criteria against which to compare student performances. These criteria are embodied in the statements of clinical objectives. The expectation is that the teacher has prepared clinical objectives for each course of study, that the clinical objectives are consistent with course objectives, and that the course objectives are appropriate to the level of study and contribute to the accomplishment of program objectives.

The clinical laboratory objectives are well known to the student and both the student and teacher plan learning activities to meet each objective. Student behaviors, then, are assessed against the stated objectives. Two important points are implied by this. First, the evaluation is done only in relation to the stated objectives. Previous learnings upon which current skill development is based are to be assumed, they are not to be reevaluated. Such skills were evaluated in a previous course and the student passed them. Only the objectives stated in a given course may be evaluated at a given time. Second, criterion referenced evaluation rather than normative evaluation is advocated in clinical judgments. Each student's performance is compared against stated behaviors in the objectives rather than against the performance of fellow classmates. The reason that criterion referenced evaluation is recommended is that in the teaching–learning process the student is striving to attain certain objectives. Individualized activities are planned to facilitate goal achievement. The focus is on the individual; the competition is with oneself as opposed to competition between and among peers. So the method used to judge performance should stress individual accomplishment with the expected level of accomplishment being the stated objectives.

The timing of such judgments is important for the teacher to consider. Each student learns at a different pace and needs to be afforded adequate time to learn. The motivation should be to learn and not to be in competition with faster learners. Yet, by a particular point, such as the end of a semester or the end of a term, all students must achieve the stated clinical objectives to progress in the program of study.

Faculty should plan for the time to teach, such as the first twelve weeks of the semester, and plan for the time to evaluate, such as the last three weeks of the semester. Students should be familiar with not only the objectives, but with the time at which learning is expected to occur and the time set aside for evaluation of such learning.

What is most important for faculty to remind themselves is that all observations of student behaviors during the "learning time" are to be utilized in a formative manner, but *not* in a summative manner. Summative remarks and judgments are to be made as a result of planned observations during the evaluation period. A student performance in the first month of a course is not to be related on the clinical evaluation sheet at the end of the semester.

With this proposed use of standards and the timing suggested for evaluation, the teacher needs to make a critical adjustment in terms of expectations of self. Specifically, the sequence of events suggested does not permit time or opportunity for data collection on every type of psychomotor skill or affective demonstration that was engaged in during the semester. Instead, sampling of performance activities of each student is of the essence.

For example, the clinical objective might be: Practices aseptic techniques in client situations. Each of the students may practice asepsis in activities such as handwashing, wound care, use of precaution techniques, and handling of sterile equipment such as in a catheterization. The teacher needs to be satisfied with sampling each student's performance in one or possibly two such activities. The sample may be drawn either selectively or at random. But other performances based on the same principles are to be assumed at the same level. Nurse faculty need to become comfortable with making a judgment on observations made of less than *all* student performances. Representative behaviors can suffice.

In both the setting of, and use of standards for evaluation, nurse faculty must be continually cognizant of the level of performance to be expected in each objective. Varying interpretations are possible not only between and among faculty teaching in the same course, but by the same faculty member at different times and even in relation to different students. But clarity in the expression of the level of the objective is essential and this was discussed in Chapter 3. Of equal importance at the time of evaluation is consistency in interpretation of the objective, and its translation as compared to expected student behaviors. Undergraduate students should be expected to perform competently; graduate students should demonstrate proficiency and mastery. Faculty discussions could profitably be spent on such differentiations. A more fair and equitable decision might be made. This is a tedious, but necessary task for teachers.

Finally, in regard to the setting of and application of standards, the matter of the perception of the student warrants some attention. Although it is generally known to nurse faculty, it perhaps needs to be keenly appreciated, that students often view the process of clinical evaluation as a threat rather than a challenge. Consequently, whenever evaluation or grading enter the scene, student behavior changes. Anxiety levels rise and creativity levels decline. The student's behavior usually moves in the direction of performing according to teacher expected behaviors. Succinctly stated, student behavior in response to evaluation looks something like the pattern shown in Figure 8.1. If this depiction of usual student behavior is appreciated and agreed upon, then the task of the faculty member is to try to reverse the above

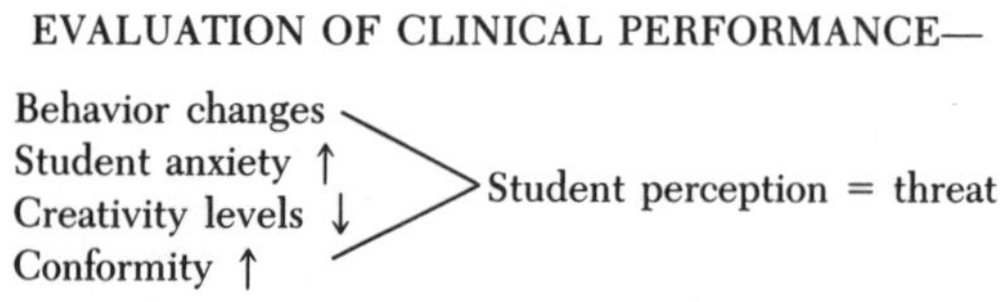

EVALUATION OF CLINICAL PERFORMANCE—

Behavior changes
Student anxiety ↑
Creativity levels ↓   > Student perception = threat
Conformity ↑

Figure 8.1 Evaluation of clinical performance.

process. The secret is to develop consistency in the teaching–learning process vis-a-vis the evaluation process. If creativity is fostered in the formative period, then creativity should be rewarded in the summative period. If students are taught to develop a sense of confidence and pride in their practice, then they will be anxious to display that confidence during the evaluation period. If "prescriptive" performances are devalued by the faculty member and individualized performances are valued, then the student becomes motivated to demonstrate nontraditional approaches to skill performance during evaluation. So the aim is to have the student's actions develop and remain consistent from the formative period through the summative period, from the learning period through the evaluation period. The goal is for the student's performance to look like that shown in Figure 8.2.

In general, the goal is for nurse faculty to foster a climate for clinical teaching and for clinical evaluation that is congruent in philosophy, standards, and reward systems. In this way, the behaviors stated in course syllabi might actually be reinforced enough to become a consistent part of the repertoire of the student's performance.

Processes

In the process of conducting clinical evaluations, the potential for increasing the validity and reliability of the judgments made is greater when multiple data sources are consulted and used. Because a number of persons are involved in the interactions constituting the clinical laboratory activities, it follows that a number of persons can and would provide data to substantiate

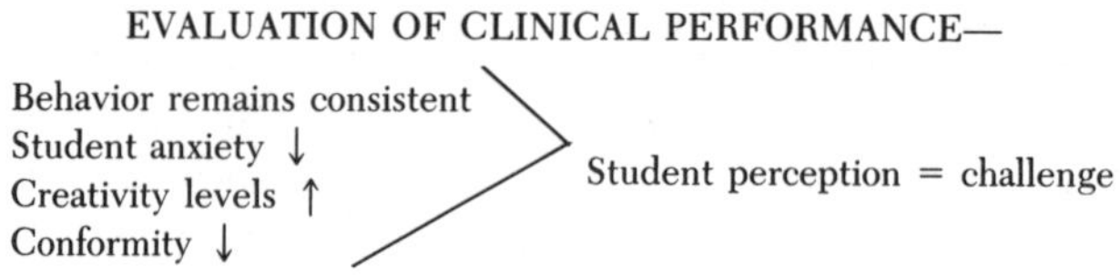

EVALUATION OF CLINICAL PERFORMANCE—

Behavior remains consistent
Student anxiety ↓
Creativity levels ↑   > Student perception = challenge
Conformity ↓

Figure 8.2 Evaluation of clinical performance.

the performance of the student. Generally, nurse faculty could broaden their data base by including data collection from these various sources. Therefore, the processes to be considered are self-evaluation, peer evaluation, client evaluation, health professional evaluation, and teacher evaluation.

If the learner has been taught to be a self-corrector, then it would follow that self-evaluation plays an important part in determining achievement. If the student knows the objectives well, and knows the behaviors expected by a given time, then that student has a major role to play, not only in working toward goal achievement, but in evaluating his or her outcomes. Given complete familiarity with the evaluation criteria, the student should write and articulate a self-evaluation. A student–teacher evaluation conference is then held to compare judgments made, explore substantiating data, and arrive at a mutal decision. In most instances, the expectation is that both the faculty member and the student will have very similar data and have arrived at very similar conclusions. The validity of the evaluation is more convincing to the student when the joint effort is made.

One of the most powerful motivators for achieving is peer pressure. Yet, this means of supporting achievement, if handled in a constructive fashion, is often overlooked. Additionally, peers possess knowledge of each others' clinical performance that can well escape the scrutiny of even the most perceptive teacher. Peers know each other well if they have been working together over a period of time. Provided that students are held strictly to the stated objectives and criteria, their shared data on each can be useful both as a motivating factor for learning and an insightful source of data for clinical evaluation. Their accountability to each other and the values of academia need to be stressed so that objectivity, fairness, and constructiveness are continually demanded. Also, in view of time constraints, the numbers of students in a clinical groups may well preclude each student doing a peer evaluation on every other student. So, methods are to be utilized to make the process manageable. For example, each student may be expected to evaluate two other students in the same clinical group. Names may be assigned through the use of a table of random numbers or through a lottery system. It may well be decided to keep confidential among the student group who is to evaluate whom. Given the desired spirit and a process that is not overly demanding of students or faculty, the process of peer evaluation can be a very valuable one.

Client evaluation is a very logical part of the process of clinical evaluation. This aspect of the evaluation process is aimed at judging the quality of the service rendered. So, this part of the process is *product-oriented*. How well did the student behaviors fulfill their intended goal when they were aimed toward client need satisfaction, that is, achievement of comfort, facilitation of mobility, relief of pain, extent of health teaching. Client evaluations can be made through informal interviews. Ask the clients how they feel after an interaction with the student; how the teaching session was of benefit; are they comfortable? Although awareness by the teacher of the *halo effect* is necessary, because some clients wish to protect the student and will rave about their performance whether or not they believe it to be the case, most are rather candid and will share honest perceptions. At any rate, the other part of client evaluation is equally important—observations made of the client by the teacher as well as review of client records. Both sources reveal outcome data related to aspects of student performance. Once again, the teacher attempts to objectify data by using the stated criteria against which to compare observations.

Other health professionals in the clinical setting who observe or interact with the students can be a valuable source of evaluation data. Staff nurses, clinical nurse specialists, physicians, pharmacists, physical therapists, dietitians, and others usually have gained insights into student performance. When asked specific questions related to the objectives, they are usually able to offer more than global generalizations. If involved in team conferences or team projects, their comments related to objectives on collaboration are imperative to faculty judgments on such activities. Health professional evaluation of students are useful on a regular basis and should be more than chance happenings.

Teacher evaluations of the student's clinical performance combine the data collected from all of the above sources together with his or her own generated data. The teacher uses the stated criteria at appropriate time to make a set of judgments regarding the accomplishment of objectives. Of course, to be able to make accurate judgments the teacher must know the student well and have had formative input into that student's development over time. The needs, motivations, goals, and aspirations of the student have been utilized in selecting clinical activities to satisy the clinical objectives. The evaluation criteria, forms, and processes are well known to the student. The various types of sources of data are also know to the student. Times for conducting the teacher's own data base are arranged with the student. After all data collection, a conference is held with each student to compare findings and judgments.

The teacher reserves the right to make the final judgment regarding student performance. This is a responsibility of teachers. Yet, broad and open processes increase the likelihood of achieving consensus with the student. The proposed system encourages checks and balances. However, even when consensus is not possible, the teacher's decision prevails with supportive data to justify it.

Tools

Any evaluation process requires paper-and-pencil guides to systematically record and weigh data. Such guides are referred to as the tools of clinical evaluation. Some tools, such as process recordings, observation logs, checklists, care plans, and videotapes are appropriate for formative evaluation. They serve as reminders of the activities and reactions to performance activities that have been accomplished and give clues as to what remains to be accomplished. Other tools are typically used in summative evaluation. Examples of such are critical incident forms, summary notes, and rating scales. In the entire process of clinical teaching and evaluation proposed in this book, the college laboratory is used extensively in formative evaluation. Study guides in the college laboratory utilized with formative tools can be assumed before the use of the clinical laboratory for each set of student activities.

Tool development appropriate to a particular program needs to proceed over a period of time. Refinement of the selected tools is to be expected through repeated usage. Also, individual faculty groups need to jointly consider and decide upon the clinical evaluation tools to be selected and used. What works well for one faculty group may very well differ from that of another faculty. One tool or a combination of tools may be used. There are, however, some basic criteria underlying useful tools:

1. The behavioral objectives determine the basis for the evaluation criteria.
2. The evaluation criteria are clearly delineated in the tool. The specific student behaviors observable only in clinical practice are explicitly stated.
3. Instructions for using the tool are carefully stated in writing for the user.
4. The same tools are used by all parties involved in the evaluation process.
5. Sample behaviors are included for each category.
6. Space is provided for recording supportive evidence.
7. Provides for natural order of sequence.
8. Space is provided for recording general statements, summaries, and recommendations.
9. Where categories are weighted for purposes of arriving at a grade, the instructions for weighting are clear and space is provided to record that weighting.

Two formats are provided by way of illustration of clinical evaluation tools. One is for formative evaluation purposes and the other is for summative purposes.

I.   Formative Evaluation Tool

Student Name _____   Course _____

Faculty Name _____   Semester _____

DIRECTIONS: For each behavior listed, circle the number that most accurately reflects the present level of performance. Use the columns to the right to record evidence of adequate learning and to specify needs for future learning.

| | Performance Scale | | | |
| | Inadequate | Adequate | | |
Desired Student Behaviors	*(−)* 3 2 1	*(+)* 1 2 3	*Adequate Learning*	*Future Learning*
1. Collects complete data base on a specific health problem.	3 2 1	1 2 3		
2. Formulates accurate nursing diagnosis in selected situations.	3 2 1	1 2 3		
3. Prioritizes nursing interventions according to client need.	3 2 1	1 2 3		

II.   Summative Evaluation Tool

Student Name _____ Course _____

Faculty Name _____ Semester _____

DIRECTIONS: Clinical objectives for this course are listed in the left-hand column. The right-hand column lists sample behaviors that would validate accomplishment of the corresponding objective. Space is also provided in this column to record actual student behaviors or activities. The column in the center provides space to check (√) if that type of activity was accomplished or not accomplished. P = accomplishment; F = nonaccomplishment. Each objective must have a P designation to achieve a *pass* on this semester's clinical activities.

Objective	P	F	Sample/Actual Behaviors
1. Conducts health teaching of clients.			Assesses need for health teaching. Uses principles of learning and teaching. Modifies teaching according to level, readiness, and motivation. (this space for recording actual behaviors)
2. Collaborates with health team members in planning and implementing client care.			Participates in health team rounds. Refers to health team members. Consults appropriate health team members. (this space for recording actual behaviors)

Grade = (Pass or Fail)

In tool #II, a point system or rating scale combined with a point system could be developed and incorporated in order to provide for a scale of more than 2 points (P-F). If, for example, a 5-point scale were preferred, the 5 points would need to be described with examples of attendant behaviors. This consideration leads to the subject of measurement.

Measurement

The subject of measurement is involved with the quantitative designation attached to a qualitative judgment of performance. The quantitative judgment is ultimately converted to a grade or symbol that is in concert with the particular institution of which the program of nursing is a part. For example, some systems require an A–F grade; others permit a P–F grade in laboratory courses. Beyond institutional policy, however, the decision as to what grade to ascribe to clinical laboratory activities remains hotly debated. There are no simple or universal answers. The subject of performance grading in and of itself is highly complex and the reader is referred to appropriate works of experts in the field of evaluation.

However, a brief consideration of this subject is included, primarily to attest to the need to make choices regarding grading systems based on the policies of the parent institution as well as on the philosophy of clinical teaching. Again, the system for clinical evaluation should be consistent with the process and spirit of clinical teaching.

For example, it would seem that with the freedom the learner, self-correction, and independence of proceeding in clinical activities ascribed to in previous chapters, that a simple two-point grading scale would support that type of learning and be congruent with the evaluative judgments that would follow. In other words, the accomplishment of objectives would either be there or not be there. The objectives would either be achieved or not achieved. Performance would either be pass or fail, acceptable or not acceptable, satisfactory or unsatisfactory.

To have more than two points on the scale would qualify performances and have the tendency to reduce creativity and restrict experimentation. The student tends to become more occupied with the grading than with the learning.

In a system with a two-point clinical performance scale and with theory or content as part of the same course, the grade earned as a result of paper-and-pencil testing (A–F) becomes the grade for the course, provided that the clinical grade was pass. If the clinical grade is fail, then the course grade is F, because in a professional field of study all teaching–learning is ultimately for the purpose of performance of the service.

On the other hand, if an A to F grading scale is supported and developed, a system of averaging the grade for paper-and-pencil testing with the clinical performance grade must be devised. Also, very importantly the specific clinical behaviors for each letter grade must be clearly delineated by the faculty group and shared with the students. For example, if an A is outstanding behavior, then outstanding behaviors must be described and a point system arrived at. The point system might appear as follows:

Categories of Behavior	Points	Sample Behaviors (based on objectives)
Outstanding behavior	4	
Above average behavior	3	
Average behavior	2	
Acceptable, but below average behavior	1	
Unacceptable behavior	0	

In clinical practice, the teacher conveys to the student the value for working toward achievement of professional behaviors first, and earning a grade second. Actually, the grade becomes a by-product of performance. But the greatest reward should be in the participation of additional varied activities and further accomplishment of desired client outcomes. If this outlook is achieved, the A–F system of grading becomes less important to the student.

Summary

Basically, what nurse faculty need to grapple with is that in clinical evaluation the behavior of the learner is likely to change in the direction of performing according to "normative" behaviors. Anxiety levels rise while creativity levels decline. Formative evaluation of practice should be nonjudgmental and provide hints and suggestions rather than criticism. Eventually, summative evaluation and grading is necessary, but it should be reserved until the end of the course of study. There should be enough time allowed to freely learn to explore without the constraints of being evaluated. Also, evaluation criteria should be directly related to specified objectives written at the level of competency for undergraduates, and at the level of proficiency and mastery for graduate students.

Notes

1. Irby, D. M., & Dohner, C. W. Student clinical performance. In Ford, C. W., & Morgan, K. (Eds). *Teaching in the health professions*. St. Louis: C. V. Mosby Company, 1976, p. 208.
2. Scriven, M. The methodology of evaluation. In *AERA monograph series in curriculum evaluation*, No. 1. Chicago: Rand McNally, 1967.
3. Dressel, P. L., & Nelson, C. H. Testing and grading policies. In Dressel, P. L. & Associates. *Evaluation in higher education*. Boston: Houghton-Mifflin Company, 1961, p. 251.

Bibliography

Benner, P., & Benner, R. *The new graduate: Perspectives, practice and promise*. La Jolla: The Coordinating Council for Education in Health Sciences for San Diego and Imperial Counties, 1975.

Bevis, E. O. *Curriculum-building in nursing*. St. Louis: C. V. Mosby Company, 1982.

Blakeney, H. *Evaluation of student achievement in associate degree nursing programs*. Unpublished doctoral dissertation, New York, Teachers College, Columbia University, 1967.

Cronin-Stubbs, D., & Mathews, J. J. A clinical performance tool for a process-oriented nursing curriculum. *Nurse Educator*, 1982, 7 (4), 24–29.

Dachelet, C. Z., Wemett, M. F., Garling, J., Craig-Kuhn, K., Kent, N., & Kitzman, H. J. The critical incident technique applied to the evaluation of the clinical practicum setting. *Journal of Nursing Education*, 1981, 20 (8), 15–31.

Department of Baccalaureate and Higher Degree Programs. *Considerations in clinical evaluation: Instructors, students, legal issues*. New York: National League for Nursing, 1979, Publication No. 16–1764.

Department of Baccalaureate and Higher Degree Programs. *The challenge of clinical evaluation*. New York: National League for Nursing, 1979, Publication No. 16–1763.

deTornyay, R. Measuring problem-solving skills by means of the simulated nursing problem test. *Journal of Nursing Education*, 1968, 7 (1), 3–8.

Dincher, J., & Stidger, S. Evaluation of a written simulation format for clinical nursing judgment. *Nursing Research*, 1976, 25 (4), 280–285.

Fivars, G., & Groenell, D. *Nursing evaluation: The problem and the process*. New York: Macmillan Book Company, 1966.

Guba, E. G., & Lincoln, Y. S. *Effective evaluation*. San Francisco, California: Jossey-Bass, 1981.

Hauser, M.A. Initiation into peer review. *American Journal of Nursing*, 1975, 75 (12), 2204–2207.

Hinshaw, A. S., & Field, M. A. An investigation of variables that underlie collegial evaluations: Peer review. *Nursing Research*, 1974, *23* (4), 292–300.

Huckabay, L., Anderson, N., & Holm, D., & Lee, J. Cognitive, affective, and transfer of learning consequences of computer-assisted instruction. *Nursing Research*, 1979, *28* (4), 228–233.

Irby, D. M., & Dohner, C. W. Student clinical performance. In Ford, C. W., & Morgan, K. (eds). *Teaching in the health professions*. St. Louis: C. V. Mosby Company, 1976.

Keeton, M. T., and Associates. *Experiential learning: Rationale, characteristics, and assessment*. San Francisco: Jossey-Bass, 1976.

Kubo, W., Chase, L., & Leton, J. A creative examination. *Nursing Outlook*, 1971, *19* (8), 524–526.

Lenburg, C. B. *The clinical performance examination*. New York: Appleton-Century-Crofts, 1979.

Litwack, L. A system for evaluation. *Nursing Outlook*, 1976, *24* (1), 45–58.

MacKay, R. C. Evaluation of faculty and students: A means toward fuller communication and greater productivity. *Journal of Nursing Education*, 1974, *13* (1)3–7.

Marcinek, S. A. *Evaluation of clinical problem solving among graduating baccalaureate nursing students using computer simulation*. Unpublished doctoral dissertation, The University of Texas at Austin, 1978.

McIntyre, J. M., McDonald, F., Bailey, J., & Claus, K. K. A simulated clinical nursing test. *Nursing Research*, 1972, *21* (5), 429–435.

Meleis, A. L., & Benner, P. Process of product evaluation? *Nursing Outlook*, 1975, *23* (4), 303–307.

Morgan, B., Luke, C., & Herbert, J. Evaluating clinical proficiency. *Nursing Outlook*, 1979, *27* (8), 540–544.

Morgan, M. K., & Irby, D. A. *Evaluating clinical competencies in the health professions*. St. Louis: C. V. Mosby Company, 1978.

Olivieri, P., & Sweeney, M. A. Evaluation of clinical learning: By computer. *Nurse Educator*, 1980, *5* (4), 26–31.

Pace, R. (ed.). *Evaluating learning and teaching*. San Francisco: Jossey-Bass, Winter (4), 1973.

Paduano, M. Evaluation in the nursing laboratory: An honest appraisal. *Nursing Outlook*, 1974, *22* (11), 702–705.

Ramphal, M. Peer review. *American Journal of Nursing*, 1974, *74* (1), 63–67.

Reilly, D. E. *Behavioral objectives—evaluation in nursing*. New York: Appleton-Century-Crofts, 1980.

Reilly, D. E. (ed.) *Teaching and evaluating the affective domain in nursing programs*. New Jersey: Charles B. Slack, Inc., 1978.

Rines, A. B. *Evaluating student progress in learning the practice of nursing*. New York: Teachers College, Columbia University, 1976.

Schneider, H. L. *Evaluation of nursing competence*. Boston: Little, Brown Co., 1979.

Scriven, M. Evaluation perspectives and procedures. In Popham, W. J. (ed.) *Evaluation in education: Current applications*. Berkeley, California: McCutchan, 1974.

Scriven, M. The methodology of evaluation. In *AERA monograph series in curriculum evaluation*. No. 1. Chicago: Rand McNally, 1967.

Simpson, J. The walk-around laboratory practical examination in evaluating clinical nursing skills. *Journal of Nursing Education*, 1967, *6* (4), 23–26.

Singer, R. N. To err to not to err: A question for the instruction of psychomotor skills. *Review of Educational Research*, 1977, *47* (3), 479–498.

Sommerfield, D. P., & Accola, K. M. Evaluating student's performance. *Nursing Outlook*, 1978, *26* (7), 432–436.

Stecchi, J. M., Woltman, S. J., Wall-Haas, C., Heggestad, B., & Zier, M. Comprehensive approach to clinical evaluation: One teaching team's solution to clinical evaluation of students in multiple settings. *Journal of Nursing Education,* 1983, *22* (1), 38–46.

Stufflebeam, D. L. Self-study of approaches to evaluation. In Popham, W. S. (Ed.). *Evaluation in education*. Berkeley, California: McCutchan Publishing Corporation, 1974.

Sumida, S. W. A computerized test for clinical decision making. *Nursing Outlook*, 1972, *20* (7), 458–461.

Sweeney, M. A., Hedstrom, B., & O'Malley, M. Process evaluation: A second look at psychomotor skills. *Journal of Nursing Education*, 1982, *21* (2), 4–17.

Wandelt, M., Stewart, D. D. *Slater nursing competencies rating scale*. New York: Appleton-Century-Crofts, 1975.

Welborn, P., & Thompson, D. Strategies for dealing with students whose clinical performance is unsatisfactory. *Journal of Nursing Education*, 1982, *21* (5), 26–30.

Wigton, R. Factors important in the evaluation of clinical performance of internal medicine residents. *Journal of Medical Education*, 1980, *55* (3), 206–208.

Wooley, A. The long and tortured history of clinical evaluation. *Nursing Outlook*, 1977, *25* (5), 308–315.

CHAPTER 9

Faculty Practice to Enhance Clinical Teaching and Research

The role expectations of the nurse faculty member have undergone a series of changes with attendant demands during the past century. From the beginnings of nursing education programs in the United States, the nurse faculty member was primarily a staff nurse who also carried responsibility for teaching students. At one point the head nurse group comprised the faculty. Then, gradually the nurse faculty were seen as being a separate group with responsibilities defined mainly in teaching. Hence, nurse faculty groups developed apart from nursing service.[1] And, of course, programs of nursing gradually moved from service institutions to institutions of higher learning.

Historically, the need to separate nursing service and nursing education to solve the problems that developed, unfortunately led to the wide gap between practitioners and educators, between caring and teaching. Lately there is a growing awareness that although up-dated knowledge and skill in a content area has been known to be essential to the effective transmission of such to students, ways must be found to assure this. In other words, "practice what you teach."[2]

And all of this is not to say that the vast majority of nurse faculty over the years have not been competent. Indeed, most faculty have been masters in the knowledge, attitudes, and skills of their area of expertise. So, what actually has been the identified problem? Interestingly, the claims of less than desired expertise have neither been studied, carefully delineated, nor documented. It would seem that the claims are at least related to maintenance of psychomotor skills, speed, dexterity, and the opportunity to test hunches regarding a practice. Also, not to be ignored is the fact that the past several years have brought an advent of rapidly changing scientific and technologic advances affecting nursing practice. It simply becomes more difficult to maintain expertise of practice without periodic involvement in it. The issues that arise surround the questions why and how?

Before addressing these questions directly, it may be well to conceptualize the historical development of the role of nurse educator as proceeding on a developmental continuum. The process of moving toward the point of maturity is reaching fruition. Nursing as a profession, as well as nursing education, is approaching maturity. Nurse faculty are becoming properly credentialed for their role in academia. Programs are educationally sound; teaching strategies are improving as far as their appropriateness to higher education. Programs of nursing are well established in the mainstream of higher education. At the same time, nursing service personnel with graduate degrees are increasing. Staff nurses with undergraduate degrees are also more prevalent. The distinct mission of nursing service to provide quality nursing service is recognized and assumed.

Although, formerly, nursing service and nursing education remained independent of each other, there is currently the need and the readiness for the two aspects of nursing, education and service, to articulate and complement each other in a way distinctively different from any previous arrangement. Rather than merge, as was the case in early years, the relationship might be one of converging in the best interests of the profession. The new relationship implies common goals and differences in responsibilities toward goal accomplishment. This suggests a new look at a number of traditional relationships between practicing nurses and nurse faculty. One of these is the role of the nurse educator regarding faculty practice. The subject of faculty practice is included here as a potential means of enhancing the faculty member's utilization of the clinical laboratory.

Faculty Member As Nurse

Many nurse faculty were conscientious, expert practitioners of nursing before becoming faculty members. Subsequently, for significant numbers of them, the intellectual as well as the emotional commitment to nursing practice continues. The struggle that ensues is related to the internalization of the role of the faculty member while maintaining the proper or expected role of the nurse.

The nurse educator who is a master of the practice of nursing can practice both intellectual and psychomotor skills as an integrated whole. Also, the spectrum of values regarding clients, students, and colleagues is very much a part of the repertoire of behaviors of this person. Prioritizing the behaviors of rendering care versus guiding learning becomes a continual, cyclic process.

Faculty Member as Teacher

The roles of a teacher in academia are clearly defined as teaching, scholarly activities, and service. Faculty practice is not a need and does not hold an established place throughout academia. So the model and its value is an elusive one.

Meeting the demands of the traditional roles of the nurse faculty member is demanding enough without the addition of faculty practice. Until quite recently the prevalent concern has been that nurse faculty may know their subject matter well, but need to focus on the transmission of the subject matter to the learner. So graduate programs include courses on teaching and learning. But the concern inherent in the issue of faculty practice seems to have switched from transmission of information to a question of the knowledge and skills to be transmitted. Indeed, the issue seems to have come full circle.

Throughout this book the nurse faculty member in the role of teacher as opposed to nurse has been supported and articulated. To fulfill the role of teacher, the often conflicting behaviors of the nurse must be put aside. To fulfill responsibilities to the university or college that is the hiring institution, time, effort, and energies need to be channeled into the role of academician. Yet, interestingly, even this latter aspect of the role is challenged in the literature. For example, two authors state, "Nurse faculty members tend to focus their energies in support of the general missions of universities: teaching, research, and community service."[3] They go on to say that there is no time for faculty practice that is much needed. But essentially, though, what person who is hired by a particular type of institution, namely an educational institution, has a right to not support its general mission?

At the same time, the argument for continuing expertise in a practice field such as nursing is not to be ignored. When facing the issue squarely, one cannot help but keenly feel the difference between liberal arts and professional faculty. The challenge is great for professional faculty. But the central mission of the faculty member cannot be overlooked. Likewise, modes of incorporating faculty practice into the total role cannot be taken lightly, prescribed, or mandated.

Faculty Member in Relation to Practice and Research

There is a relationship between knowing how to practice and knowing how to improve practice. If the faculty member is a master practitioner, then

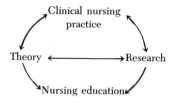

Figure 9.1 Complement of education and practice.

utilization of practice opportunities should also be geared to improving the quality of practice in a given area. In turn, the concern with improved quality of practice has direct implications for the teaching of nursing. Quality practice enhances quality teaching.

The entire approach to "what is nursing practice" is undergoing scrutiny. Teaching strategies are moving in a direction such that the transmission of factual information is kept to a minimum and the conceptualization involving use of theory to guide practice is maximized. Because the field of nursing is one of applied science, the research findings of a number of scientific fields determine the approach to nursing assessment, underlie our plans, guide our interventions, and suggest questions for evaluation. Careful analysis of outcomes lead to research findings in nursing and the subsequent development of nursing theory. The point is that theory must guide practice and practice must be used to generate theory (see Figure 9.1). The nurse faculty member could contribute much to this total process through engaging in practice. Also, such theoretic explorations lead to a substantially different approach to clinical teaching, namely, the view should be that all of clinical laboratory is an experiment. All clinical laboratory activities involve the manipulation of variables. All clinical laboratory activities generate hypotheses.

Contrast of Behaviors of Nurse Versus Nurse Educator

As the subject of faculty practice is pursued, it seems important to keep in mind that the learned behaviors of the nurse not only differ from those of the nurse educator, but may be in conflict with them. When a nurse becomes a nurse educator, if this difference is realized and if there is a true interest in fully pursuing the role of educator, then a change of behavior is gradually accomplished. The educator shifts from a focus on the needs of the client to the needs of the learner. Subsequently, as the interest in faculty practice develops, these very same differences in behaviors need to be recollected and serve as a guide for decision making and planning. The teaching behav-

TABLE 9.1. Behaviors of Nurse vs. Nurse Educator

Practicing Nurse	*Nurse Educator*
Renders total care	Facilitates students' discovery of how to give aspects of care
Practices in one setting	Guides students through a wide variety of settings
Conducts prescriptive health teaching	Allows students the freedom to explore learning
Conducts evaluation of care with client input	Guides students to determine own level of accomplishment
Role model of nurse	Role model of teacher

iors should not change; the aim of the faculty member actually becomes one of adding to the dimension to the faculty role, of which one dimension is teacher. Table 9.1 considers a few such behaviors.[4]

Major differences in the use of the clinical laboratory face the practitioner and the educator. As a practitioner of nursing the clinical laboratory serves as a place within which to render quality care. As a nurse educator the clinical laboratory is a place where a nursing student comes in contact with clients and families for the purpose of acquiring intellectual and psychomotor skills. The nurse is comfortable with and proceeds from an integration of knowledge and skills; the nurse educator needs to proceed as a teacher to provide for initial, partial task learning in selected settings before providing for and expecting integrative performances. The nurse focuses on the individual needs of the client; the nurse educator focuses on the individual needs of the student while allowing the student to discover client needs.

Because the behaviors are widely differing ones, it becomes obvious that they cannot be practiced simultaneously. Perhaps the issue of faculty practice is not one of whether or not to practice, but points up the need to practice these sets of behaviors separately—at different times and in different places. Then the benefit of one set of behaviors can be realized in the practice of the other set of behaviors.

Why Faculty Practice?

Faculty practice has led to the development of a number of arguments in support as well as against the subject. There is little agreement regarding its its benefits; there is far from universal agreement regarding how it might best be arranged within a faculty member's priorities and schedule. The following discussion summarizes some of the pros and cons of faculty practice. It is included primarily as a means of considering what the appropriateness of this activity might be as it relates to all of the former discussion of the proposed role of the nurse faculty member in clinical teaching.

Arguments for Faculty Practice. The most widely proposed argument for faculty practice is that it is needed to maintain clinical skills. This is believed to be particularly important for faculty who teach courses with a clinical component. Obviously, the implication is that the exposure to clinical practice necessitated through clinical teaching is not sufficient to remain current in a field. The call is for nurse faculty to practice nursing apart from their teaching.

Another prevalent supportive argument is that regular clinical practice on the part of nurse educators is important to establishing credibility with groups who interact with this faculty member, namely, students, practitioners of nursing, health team members, and clients. The thrust of this argument is to *prove* that one *can* do as they preach. Together with established credibility, faculty practice is said to provide high quality care to clients and thereby improve the quality of care rendered in the setting. This argument flows from the belief that the best prepared, most expert practitioners leave practice for education; nursing service and the health care system is thereby deprived of the potential benefits of such high quality care if the faculty member does not practice. Documentation of the provision of such care and its benefits to clients could serve as data to support legislation on third party payments to nurses.

Also, faculty practice is proposed to enhance the faculty role by improving teaching and providing a source of ideas for scholarly activities. In the realm of teaching, ongoing clinical practice is believed to suggest client illustrations and case studies for exploration with students. Additionally, research questions are generated through continued practice in a specialized area. So research and practice are expected to be closely linked. Not only would such facilitation of research projects benefit the faculty member in promotion and tenure decisions in academia, but the practitioner as researcher is a desirable role model for students.

Arguments against Faculty Practice. Equally vociferous are those who emphasize the cons of faculty practice. Those on this side of the issue contend that clinical activities with students are sufficient to keep abreast of practice in their area of expertise. Furthermore, the argument contends that psychomotor skills are too readily lost if not practiced on a regular basis, and that the nurse educator cannot practice enough to maintain optimal skills. Additionally, there is the related question as to whether or not the performance of clinical skills has any relationship to the quality of teaching. Some very effective teachers do not possess high levels of skill performance. It does not require clinical skills to convey concepts. Instead it requires teaching skills.

Those opposed to faculty practice also offer that there is insufficient time in a faculty member's schedule to allow for such regular practice. Heavy teaching loads, committee work, service projects, writing research, consultation, and giving papers present already ominous demands on time and energy without the seriously heavy demands of practice. It is believed that involvement in faculty practice would actually drain time from scholarly productivity, thus compounding the problem of large numbers of faculty in lower ranks that has been a nagging problem in schools and departments of nursing for many years. Suggested times for practice have been semester breaks, summers, and sabbatical leaves, which detracts from time otherwise spent in research and writing by other faculty, still leaving the nurse faculty members at a disadvantage.

Another set of objections arise from what may be termed a lack of readiness of academia to administer and reward for faculty practice. There are no standards for designing effective models of faculty practice and, thus, no standards for evaluation of faculty practice. For example, is faculty practice to consist of hands on care? Is consultation to nurse colleagues in clinical settings considered faculty practice? Does faculty practice mean carrying a regular caseload? If so, 24-hour availability is assumed with "on call" responsibility. Or, is faculty practice the management of a nursing unit and nursing personnel? Parameters of practice are unclear. Additionally, regardless of the nature of the service and the time required to deliver it, there is no system of credit for faculty practice in academia. Credit toward achievement of tenure or promotion as well as monetary achievement remains elusive.

The benefits of regular faculty practice are questioned. For those striving to be role models of teachers as opposed to nurses, faculty practice could serve to heighten role conflict as one switches from one role to the other. Such role conflict could be evidenced if the same clinical settings are used for teaching and practice. Instead, these opponents advocate the use of clinical preceptors to serve as the role model of the nurse. Finally, in this area of benefits, there is no documented evidence that faculty practice improves the quality of care in institutions or that faculty practice improves performance as a teacher. This evidence is absent despite some faculty practice models that have been in place for some years.

Opponents of faculty practice fear a work overload for nurse educators with the addition of such a weighty responsibility that could result in burnout. Coupled with that is the concern that practice could, for some, serve as a legitimized escape from developing in the faculty role as set forth by academia.

Approaches to Incorporating Practice
into the Faculty Role

The issue of faculty practice requires systematic study and deliberation by nurse faculty. It is an issue that will not go away in the near future. The arguments pro and con each provide points that merit serious consideration. Problems abound in envisioning such practice. Existing models are limited to a small group of nurse educators, namely the practitioner–teacher model, joint appointments, released time for practice, and collaborative practice arrangements. Limited success has been demonstrated by any one of them. No satisfactory reimbursement plans exist, either to the individual faculty member or the institution. The scarcity of third party reimbursement mechanisms for nurses additionally complicates the situation. Medical faculty models are thus unsatisfactory as comparisons. Also, medical faculty can practice and spend much less time with their clients than nurses need to spend.

The time element is not to be ignored. Where might the time for practice come from? Other related considerations are travel time, space, and secretarial assistance. And finally, there is the difficulty of assuring recognition for faculty practice by the rest of the university. How might there be differentiation of expectations among ranks? How will the activity fit in with criteria for promotion, tenure, and reappointment?

There are no clear-cut, easy, or universal solutions to the problems regardless of one's position on the central issue. But what seems important is that there be flexibility in terms of practice expectations of nurse faculty. Some may need to and want to practice, others may not. To impose a demand on all nurse faculty is dangerous and pointless. The particular expertise of each faculty member is to be used to advantage—and talents vary widely.

Testing of models for faculty practice in a systematized fashion is imperative. Incorporate an evaluation plan into each model. Project data is most convincing. Also, within these models, the choice of setting, clientele, and clinical activities should be reserved to the faculty member. Otherwise, one might truly question the motivation for, and the potential benefits of faculty practice. Is it another of a series of attempts by nurses to be all things to all people? Is it but a continuation of the striving to be perfect beyond human possibility? Such thoughts have been well articulated by McCarthy[5]:

> The quest for perfection has a long and venerable history within the profession of nursing. . . In the sixties we pinned our hopes on clinical nurse specialists; later, on nurse practitioners. The current victims of our unsatisfied need are nurse faculty . . . that nurse faculty engage regularly in clinical practice. . . It is more likely that each of the arguments in support

of faculty practice is a rationalization of that powerful unconscious wish to be perfect. Consider though, that if nursing would allow itself to be less than perfect, it would then be exactly equal, on that score alone, to every other profession."

Summary

It may well become important for nurse faculty to engage in practice to increase their practice skills and orientation to practice. Their practice could serve as the source of their research problems as well as a source of clients for their teaching. Indeed, the ideal interfacing between practice, research, and education could be most aptly demonstrated by and through nurse educators.

However, analysis of this challenge of faculty practice to date, leads to the inference that faculty practice be pursued apart from, rather than integrated with, the role of teacher. Basically, it is believed and maintained that faculty members should be role models of teachers, not of nurses, and that they should be deeply involved in teaching as opposed to providing care. The two roles require widely differing sets of behaviors that are in many respects in direct opposition to each other. Therefore, one person cannot behave according to the two role sets simultaneously. Yet, when taken separately, in separate contexts, the two roles can, at least theoretically, benefit the repertoire of behaviors useful to the one person.

So, the need for faculty to practice will continue to be debated, but such practice should be considered apart from the time when the faculty member is teaching. Perhaps on a given day each week; or a given period during the year when school is not in session. Various models could be tested that would fit the individual belief system of schools. Also, not to be lost in all of this is the individuality of faculty. Different faculty members bring to our faculties different strengths; let us capitalize on them and reward them. Hopefully we can avoid the disaster that could result from the expectation that all faculty should practice according to the same model. Indeed, some faculty may not practice, and instead make their contributions in other ways. It is the richness of diversity among faculty members that leads to a high quality faculty.

The subject of faculty practice inherently has very demanding responsibilities—added to already existing heavy responsibilities. Although a timely issue with reasonably good benefits to be gained, the caution is to strike a balance in total career demands. For there is nothing to gain in the field and everything to lose from leading our members to burnout.

Notes

1. Dolan, J. A., Fitzpatrick, M. L., & Herrmann, E. K. *Nursing in society: A historical perspective.* Philadelphia: W. B. Saunders Company, 1983, pp. 171–189.
2. Machan, L. *The practitioner-teacher role: Practice what you teach.* Wakefield, Mass.: Nursing Resources, 1980.
3. Collison, C. R., & Parsons, M. A. Is practice a viable faculty role? *Nursing Outlook,* 1980, *28* (11),677.
4. Infante, M. S. Nurse vs. nurse educator: Conflicting roles for the teacher of nursing. *Nursing Outlook.* In press for 1985.
5. McCarthy, P. Editorial. Will faculty practice make perfect? *Nursing Outlook,* 1981, *29* (3), 163.

Bibliography

Bracken, R., & Christman, L. An incentive program designed to reward clinical competence.*Journal of Nursing Administration, 1978, 10* (1), 8–18.

Brykczynski, F., Hayes, W. S., Waters, L. D., et al. Nursing faculty develop primary care skills. *Nursing and Health Care,* 1981, *2* (10), 538–542.

Chickadonz, G., Bush, E. G., Korthuis, K. E., & Utz, S. W. Mobilizing faculty toward integration of practice into faculty roles. *Nursing and Health Care,* 1981, *2* (10), 548–553.

Christy, T. E. Clinical practice as a function of nursing education: An historical analysis. *Nursing Outlook,* 1980, *28* (8), 493–497.

Collison, C. R., & Parsons, M. A. Is practice a viable faculty role? *Nursing Outlook,* 1980, *28* (11), 677–679.

Dinsmore, V., & Pollow, R. Credit for faculty practice model: A proposal. *Nursing and Health Care,* 1981, *2* (1), 17–21.

Holm, K. Faculty practice—Noble intentions gone awry? *Nursing Outlook,* 1981, *29* (11), 655–657.

Keen, M. F., & Dear, M. R. Mastery of role transition: Clinical teaching strategies. *Journal of Nursing Education,* 1983, *22* (5), 183–186.

Kellmer, D. M. The lack of effective faculty role models within professional schools. *Nursing and Health Care,* 1982, *31* (1), 44–45, 54.

Machan, L. *The practitioner–teacher role: Practice what you teach.* Wakefield, Mass.: Nursing Resources, 1980.

Mariano, C. H. *Perceptions of baccalaureate nursing faculty regarding the primary source and primary means of their learning to teach students selected processes of nursing*. Unpublished doctoral dissertation, Teachers College, Columbia University, 1978.

Mauksch, I. G. Faculty practice: A professional imperative. *Nurse Educator*, 1980, 5 (3), 21–24.

McCarthy, P. A. Editorial. Will faculty practice make perfect? *Nursing Outlook*, 1981, *29* (3), 163.

Smith, G. R. Compensating faculty for their clinical practice. *Nursing Outlook*, 1980, *28* (11), 673–676.

Wakefield-Fisher, M. The issue: Faculty practice. *Journal of Nursing Education*, 1983, *22* (5), 207–210.

CHAPTER 10

The Challenge
of Clinical Teaching
for Nurse Educators

The previous discussions of the nature of clinical teaching in nursing education, suggested strategies for teaching in the college and clinical laboratory, clinical evaluation, and the brief exploration of some role-related issues for nurse faculty who teach in clinical laboratories support the complexity of the process of clinical teaching. And, because of this complexity, fulfilling the responsibility adequately can be both fatiguing and overwhelming. To maintain this view as a threat to, or loss of, the desired academic functioning of the nurse educator can only lead to burnout and loss of valuable people in faculty ranks.

Instead, the exciting challenge of clinical laboratory teaching can be sensed through a rethinking and newly designed use of the clinical settings for students. The essential elements can serve as a useful guide. Gradually, various approaches to clinical teaching can be tested for their usefulness in various educational programs. Unique approaches to the clinical laboratory can be experimented with and developed to replace traditional uses that have proved unsatisfactory. What is basic to such experimentation is to keep sight of the nature and purpose of the clinical laboratory in nursing education. And the incentive to put forth the effort required is the constant realization that the nurse educator can not only change the way nursing is taught, but can ultimately change the way nursing is practiced.

In an attempt to accomplish these changes, the following discussion will consider the role of the nurse educator in nursing and nursing education, a view of the behaviors to be exhibited by nurse educators, and a realization of the challenge inherent in clinical teaching.

176

Role of the Nurse Educator in Nursing and Nursing Education

It might well be said that nurse educators are responsible for the quality of the practice of nursing that has occurred in the past, and is currently in evidence, as well as for that which might be in the future. It is the educators who mold the behaviors that are expected to persist over the duration of a career. And when these desired practice behaviors are not evident, either because they are not practiced consistently over time or because they are not valued by our graduates, the blame is usually placed on the constraints imposed by clinical settings. Although, to some extent that may be true, it might also be true that the opportunity to develop these desired practices was not provided consistently during the educational program. If approaches to the use of clinical settings were creatively designed and utilized by nurse faculty, and if the opportunities for truly professional practice were enjoyed by nursing students, the products of nursing programs would understand what quality practice is and feel a commitment to contribute to the development of a climate for that practice to occur in nursing service.

Clearly, the challenge for nurse educators is to prepare practitioners who have *acquired* the professional behaviors articulated in program objectives; the challenge is to have inculcated values for quality practice for clients; the challenge is to graduate professional nurses who would not dream of practicing otherwise. This set of expectations requires a change in behaviors on the part of nurse faculty in clinical teaching.

Through such changes, the nurse faculty member would offer nursing students the same level and type of learning activities that other university and college students enjoy in laboratory courses. In turn, the faculty member would enjoy the same rewards of the teaching process that other university and college faculty enjoy. Beyond the educational program, nurse faculty could look forward to nurses taking the rightful place of prestige and respect within the health care delivery system. The role of the nurse educator in reshaping the image of nurses into professionals and in influencing the direction of nursing practice toward high quality would become a reality. All of this is for educators to produce, and for students, clients, and other health professionals to enjoy.

But to become a reality, nurse faculty must have a vision of what that practice is, and be willing to test alternative strategies in clinical teaching to prepare the nurses who will deliver that practice. Florence Nightingale appreciated the need for change in nursing education. Her words are a fitting reminder for nurse educators today:

> For us who nurse, our nursing is a thing which, unless in it we are making progress every year, every month, every week, take my word for it, we are

going back. The more experience we gain, the more progress we can make . . . After all, all that our training can do for us is teach us how to train ourselves.[1]

Quest for Change in Behaviors of Nurse Educators

The transition from the role of nurse to nurse educator is not an easy or natural metamorphosis. It is only recently that recognition and attention have been duly given to the socialization process that systematically guides a nurse to move from the role of care-giver to that of facilitator of the learning of the knowledges and skills that underlie caregiving.[2] However, in moving from the role of nurse to nurse educator, commitment to the care-giving role is not easy for nurses to put aside intellectually or emotionally. And often, the priority commitment to caregiving persists to the detriment of the learning of students.

Also to be considered is the premise that becoming a nurse educator is also not an additive process, that is, the addition of the role of educator to that of nurse. Rather, it requires a shift in knowledge, skills, behaviors, and values that prepare a nurse for newly assimilated roles, settings, and goals shared by new reference groups.[3] A resocialization process is needed during graduate study leading to teacher prepation. During this socialization process a number of key behaviors formerly acquired and practiced change. Although role conflict and role confusion can be expected to be experienced in varying degrees at various times, such conflict can be greatly reduced through an intellectualization of the difference between the practice role and the teaching role.

Without such a clear differentiation and the development of attendant behaviors, the nurse educator poises herself for burnout. And that burnout can occur for either or both of two reasons. First, as a result of the process of socialization into nursing, nurses believe that they must satisfy all needs for all clients. The extension of this notion into nursing education translates into the perceived mandate that faculty must teach all there is to know about nursing to all students. In the words of Jeglin-Mendez[4] we go". . . right on with the impossible pattern, exhausting ourselves attempting to instruct and evaluate the 'whole.' We also were committed to the unwritten code of the-student-must-know-this-before-they-graduate." The resocialization process requires that nurse educators use broad concepts and sample behaviors optimally to teach the knowledge, skills, and attitudes of nursing.

The second reason for burnout surrounds the lack of role change and role clarity for the faculty role. Confusing the role of nurse with the role of faculty member leads to tension and frustration. Role clarity requires that the roles be appropriately separated and that the teacher understand that he or she is a faculty member whose content area is nursing. "For the clinician it is the client who commands her expert ability; for the academician it is the student."[5] In trying to do both, the faculty member will experience what Conway and Glass call "discovery overload syndrome." This eventually leads to burnout due to an inability to control and monitor workload and no attempt to negotiate role demands.

Through a systematic process of preparation of nurse educators for these possibilities, some role conflict can be averted and some can be managed in order to avert a crisis. Conflict resolution is based on the broadened understanding of the differentiation between the role of nurse and the role of educator.

An outcome of equal importance in this process of socialization is the expectation that role clarity will lead to enhanced role fulfillment as a faculty member. Nurse faculty would have more energy to devote to scholarly productivity and become full-fledged members of academia. Except for the noteworthy achievements of a relatively small number of nurse faculty, fulfillment of all aspects of the faculty role remains elusive. For many are pursuing credentialing plus attempting to produce in the area of scholarship. Armiger[6] states that nursing education has won admission to academe but, for full acceptance its professors must meet the same expectations for scholarly productivity, especially with respect to research and publications, as their colleagues in other disciplines.

The faculty role in practice could develop appropriately according to the guidelines presented in Chapter 9. Interest in and contributions to practice need not be abandoned; complementary roles could be developed. However, for the novice faculty member, simultaneous role acting may be stressful. A sequential approach to dual role development might proceed as suggested by Barley and Redman.[7] They conceptualize the continuum of development to a full faculty role as passing from single role awareness (teacher), to full role functioning, to the ability to move easily within several roles frequently and simultaneously. Such a progression may lead to eventual quadradic role fulfillment of teacher, scholar, leader, and practitioner. It may better meet the expectations of academicians as well as practitioners. But through separate role playing, it may also better meet the needs of students of nursing.

Realizing the Opportunity Inherent in Clinical Teaching

Nurse educators alone carry the primary responsibility for preparing the practitioners of nursing of tomorrow. The manner in which they will practice will be highly correlated with the type of clinical activities they engaged in as students. These nurses will practice as they have been taught. Testing of creative approaches to learning to practice in clinical settings is essential for nurse educators.

The society of consumers of nursing care are increasing in affluence, demands, and expectations. They expect quality care at a reasonable cost. Additionally, legislation regarding third party reimbursement for nurses and diagnostic related groups used by hospitals is increasing the demand for nursing services. More nurses will be in greater contact with clients and in more varied settings. The opportunity for that needed change in the image of nurses among consumers is ripe; educators need to prepare practitioners to behave accordingly. Nurse educators must produce highly competent practitioners who can develop sound professional judgment, and this must be done while maximizing scarce resources. The challenge is indeed great, but nursing can accomplish much by meeting that challenge.

As for the nurse educators themselves, scholarly productivity can no longer be excused. "The time has come" to have doctorally prepared faculty engaged in research and publication along with the other academicians. To be productive and meet the demands of teaching, vastly different approaches to clinical laboratory must be developed. A scholar's approach to practice and teaching is essentially what is called for. Greater consistency of approaches between teaching strategies and scholarly activities would result in reduced tension, less role conflict, and greater productivity.

Professions will always be faced with the dilemma of how to provide quality programs while keeping costs down; with producing practitioners competent to meet current and future needs while keeping tuition costs within reason; and to prepare for tomorrow's practice without losing sight of today's demands and resources. These points will require continual reexamination. There is a need for openness and creativity on the subject. There are ways through which nurse educators can better accomplish the goals of nursing education. It is not adequate to teach as one has been taught.

Nurse faculty might benefit from careful scrutiny of the implications for nursing education in the description of the educational mission of Yale by its President, Bartlett Giamatti: "Not to make one technically or professionally proficient, but to instill some sense of love of learning for its own sake, some capacity to analyze any issue as it comes along, the capacity to think and to express the results of one's thinking clearly, regardless of what the subject matter might be."[8] As we approach the twenty-first century the mandate is the same for professionals. The only difference is that professionals must also possess psychomotor skills.

> There are no perfect and complete solutions to the problems we face in teaching in the clinical laboratory. And no single formula will work well in

every setting. Yet, the clinical laboratory is so vital a part of nursing education that we can no longer rely on traditional teaching methods that appear riddled with problems for students, faculty, and consumers. No excuses can justify perpetuating the problems of yesterday and today into tomorrow."9

Notes

1. Nightingale, F. *Florence Nightingale to her nurses*. New York: The Macmillan Co., 1914.
2. Mauksch, I. G. The socialization of nurse faculty. *Nurse Educator*, 1982, 7 (4), 7.
3. Infante, M. S. Nurse vs. nurse educator: Conflicting roles for the teacher of nursing. *Nursing Outlook*. In press for 1985.
4. Jeglin-Mendez, A. M. Burnout in nursing education. *Journal of Nursing Education*, 1982, 21 (4), 30.
5. Conway, M. E., & Glass, L. K. Socialization for surviving in the academic world. *Nursing Outlook*, 1978,26 (7), 424–429.
6. Armiger, B. Scholarship in nursing. *Nursing Outlook*. 1974, 22 (3), 160–164.
7. Barley, Z., & Redman, K. Faculty role development in university schools of nursing. *Journal of Nursing Administration*, 1979, 9 (5), 43–47.
8 *New York Times Magazine*, March 20, 1983, p.42.
9. Infante, M. S. Toward effective and efficient use of the clinical laboratory. *Nurse Educator*, 1981, 6 (1), 16.

Bibliography

Argyris, C., & Schön, D. A. *Theory in practice: Increasing professional effectiveness*. San Francisco: Jossey-Bass Publishers, 1977.

Batey, M. V. The two normative worlds of the university nursing faculty. *Nursing Forum*, 1969, 7 (1), 4–16.

Fawcett, J. Integrating research into the faculty workload. *Nursing Outlook*, 1979, 27 (4), 259–262.

Henry, J. K. Nursing and tenure. *Nursing Outlook*, 1981, 29 (4), 240–244.

Jeglin-Mendez, A. M. Burnout in nursing education. *Journal of Nursing Education*, 1982, 21 (4), 29–34.

Kohnke, M. *Advocacy: Risk and reality*. St. Louis: C. V. Mosby Co., 1982.

Lillard, J. The socialization process: A student's viewpoint. *Nurse Educator*, 1982, 7 (4), 11–12.

Mauksch, I. G. The socialization of nurse-faculty. *Nurse Educator*, 1982, 7 (4), 7–10.

Mauksch, I. G., & Miller, M. H. *Implementing change in nursing*. St. Louis: C. V. Mosby Co., 1981.

Mullane, M. K. *Nursing faculty roles and functions in the large university setting*. Memo to Members: Council of Baccalaureate and Higher Degree Programs, New York: National League for Nursing, 1969.

Ozimek, D., & Yura, H. *Considerations for the effective utilization of nursing faculty in baccalaureate and higher degree programs*. New York: National League for Nursing Publication, 1977. Publication No. 15–1655.

Redman, B. Conflicts in clinical teaching in nursing. *Nursing Forum*, 1965, 4 (2), 48–53.

APPENDIX

Summary of Study of the Clinical Laboratory

This appendix presents a summary of the research conducted for the purpose of assessing the use of the clinical laboratory in nursing education as it actually existed at the time. The study was an attempt aimed at determining if and to what extent the essential elements of the clinical laboratory as already presented were, in fact, embodied in clinical laboratory activities in nursing education. Although a cursory review of the elements might lead a number of nurse educators to conclude that they might have been aware of these elements and have incorporated them into their clinical teaching, a closer examination of their activities and the activities of their students in this setting may demonstrate that this view is not entirely true. It is possible that the elements could be taken for granted. A systematic investigation of each on the part of faculty members clearly point up where the strengths as well as the shortcomings exist.

The data presented show that the vast majority of nurse educators believe in the importance of each element but how, in many instances, they failed to practice them. The presentation of such data could well serve to lead many faculty members to identify reasons why this happens to be the case and to determine how it might be altered. The elements may well serve to provide a framework from which to judge the direction of clinical laboratory activities. They could serve as a model on which to base future planning for clinical laboratory activities.

This study was undertaken to determine to what extent the clinical laboratory activities in selected baccalaureate programs in nursing embody the essential elements of the laboratory concept. The purposes of the study were to identify the essential elements of the laboratory concept; to determine the current practices engaged in by teachers of nursing in the clinical laboratory; to examine the clinical laboratory activities in baccalaureate education in nursing in light of the essential elements of a clinical laboratory; and to utilize findings as a guide for teachers in planning clinical laboratory activities for nursing students in baccalaureate programs.

The study is descriptive in nature. The laboratory concept served as a theoretical framework for this study. The essential elements of the laboratory concept evolved as a result of a search of the literature on the subject. Literature on laboratory teaching methods, and techniques in general were reviewed, as well as writings on the use of the laboratory in educational programs. Particular attention was paid to the clinical laboratory in the professions. However, the professions that were examined were limited to nursing, teaching, medicine, and social work. It is believed that similar findings would have resulted from a consideration of other professions, because similarities among those examined were readily apparent.

Assumptions

The assumptions that underlie this study are three. First, laboratory activities are an integral part of the total curriculum in education for the professions. Second, students' activities in the clinical laboratory are the crucial part of the total laboratory experience. Third, teachers provide opportunity for laboratory activities for students in light of their own perceptions of a laboratory concept.

Limitations

Data collection in this study is limited to the fourteen elements of the laboratory concept identified. This number is not intended to be interpreted as exhaustive.

Also, because the sample was drawn from the population of nurse educators in baccalaureate programs in New England, the findings can be generalized to that population only.

Development of the Instrument

The instrument that was used to collect the data was a self-administered, mail questionnaire. The intent of the questionnaire was to determine the beliefs and current practices engaged in by teachers in the clinical laboratory in selected baccalaureate programs in nursing.

The questions were constructed by using the essential elements or major characteristics of the clinical laboratory. Each question was formulated by using the theoretic components of each of the essential elements as discussed in Chapter 3. The postulated range of variations, which is a modification of the Kluckhohn-Strodtbeck Model[1] for the Classification of Basic Value Orientations, was used to develop the three possible responses to each of the multiple-choice questions. A response was developed for each of the three variations. Each response was designed to reflect the laboratory concept, mixture concept, or worker concept.

The questionnaire consisted of three parts. The first part was for the purpose of collecting personal data. This data provided a set of variables through which to view and analyze responses. In the analysis, the age, education, faculty rank, types of experiences, and area of specialization in nursing are examined to determine how these variables affect the way faculty respond to the questions. The second part contained the "belief items," which relate to what the faculty members believe laboratory activities in baccalaureate nursing education should include, or what faculty members say that they do in the clinical laboratory. The third part contained the "do items," which relate to what the respondents actually do in given situations in the clinical laboratory.

The multiple-choice items have three choices. The one choice respresented the laboratory concept wherein the principles of sound educational practice as established for the questionnaire are operational. A second choice represented the worker-oriented approach to teaching in the clinical laboratory. Emphasis on accomplishing tasks is evident. The tasks referred to are those that are ordinarily performed by a nurse practitioner or auxiliary nurse personnel and not by a student learning to become a practitioner of nursing. A third choice was a mixture. It states activities that represent some aspects of the laboratory concept and some aspects of the worker-oriented approach to teaching. The series of questions asked were a sample of all the kinds of questions that could have been asked. They were intended to get at a representative selection of teaching situations that could reflect the laboratory concept, the mixture concept, and the worker concept. The questions were designed not to get at the way a particular situation is handled, but instead to get at the way a type of situation is handled. The three choices were randomized by alphabetizing them for each question.

Attention was given to determining the validity of the items on the questionnaires. The basic issue focused on whether or not the instrument measured what it was intended to measure. Content validity was used to determine the representativeness or sampling adequacy of the content of the items. The judgments of the faculty member and graduate students who participated in the preliminary testing of the instrument, as well as the reactions of other doctoral candidates knowledgeable in the content area, were sought and used in the construction of the final draft of the questionnaire. In the determination of the content validity, the essential elements, their major components, and the postulated range of variations implied in the alternative responses constituted the basis for their judgment.

Sample

Selection of Baccalaureate Programs.   The study population consisted of teachers of nursing in senior colleges and universities in New England that provide programs of baccalaureate education in nursing. Twenty such programs in New England were listed by the New England Council on Higher Education for Nursing and were considered for participation . It was decided to restrict participant schools to those who had graduated at least one class so that faculty members might answer the questions in relation to a course that they were currently teaching. Subsequently, fourteen schools qualified for participation in the study.

Requests for Participation.   The deans, directors, or chairpersons of the fourteen baccalaureate programs in nursing in New England who had graduated at least one class were contacted and requested to permit their faculty to participate in the study. A form was enclosed for their convenience to secure demographic data on the schools, as well as to obtain a list of the names of eligible faculty members and their area of clinical specialization. Eleven of the fourteen schools agreed to participate and returned the form. The total population of nurse faculty in these schools numbered 272 and it was this population that was studied.

Procedure in Data Collection.   Each of the faculty members was contacted by mail. In the letter, faculty members were requested to participate in the study by answering the questions on the enclosed questionnaire. The letter indicated that the administrator of their school had granted permission for the school to participate in the project. In most instances faculty had already signified to the dean their willingness to participate.

After completing the questionnaire, the faculty member was requested to return the questionnaire in the enclosed stamped, self-addressed envelope. Because the questionnaire was anonymous, each participant also was requested to return the self-addressed enclosed postcard on which his or her name and school had been typed to signify that she had mailed the questionnaire.

The Participating Schools.   Eleven baccalaureate schools of nursing in New England participated in the study. The schools varied in size from a student enrollment of 124 students to an enrollment of 543 students. The size of the faculty teaching in the baccalaureate program ranged from ten to 70 teachers. The two youngest schools were five years old, and the oldest school was 28 years old.

All of the participating programs offered clinical nursing courses in the junior and senior years of the student's program. Eight of the schools offered clinical nursing courses in the sophomore year, as well as in the junior and senior years. Of the remaining three schools, two offered such courses only in the junior and senior year; one offered these courses in all four years of the program.

The Participating Faculty Members.   Each of the participants in the study was a nurse teaching in a baccalaureate program in nursing education in New England. Each was currently teaching in a course that had a clinical laboratory. Three of the returned questionnaires were returned unanswered. Two of these respondents wrote that they were not teaching in clinical nursing courses; one person replied that the questionnaire was inappropriate to her course. One hundred eighty-seven questionnaires were returned. One hundred eighty-four, or 81 percent of the entire sample, returned completed questionnaires that were included in the analysis of the data.

Of the 227 faculty members contacted, 114 were listed as having a clinical area of specialization in medical-surgical nursing; 36 in public health nursing; 47 in maternal-child health nursing; and 30 in mental health and psychiatric nursing.

Findings

Expressed Beliefs of Faculty Concerning Clinical Laboratory.   For the most part, faculty expressed the belief that the essential elements that were surveyed should be operating in the clinical laboratory activities in nursing education. In 12 of 19 instances, more than 90 percent of the sample expressed a positive belief that corresponded to the laboratory concept in regard to each particular element. In two instances, in response to questions on critical thinking and professional judgment, 100 percent of the respondents replied in the affirmative.

More than 90 percent of the faculty members responded positively to the belief that the following essential elements should be operating in the clinical laboratory: patient contact, guidance of the learner to function independently, individuation of activities, intellectual skill learning, critical thinking, problem solving, observation, experimentation, professional judgment, and transfer of knowledge. As many as 86.41 percent believed that the clinical laboratory activities in which students in their course engaged in developed their creative abilities. In the area of skill learning, more respondents believed that the clinical laboratory provided the student with the opportunity to develop intellectual skills (99.45 percent) than with the opportunity to develop motor skills (86.95 percent).

One hundred fifteen respondents, or 62 percent, expressed the belief that, to accomplish the objectives of their course, the clinical laboratory hours should remain unchanged. Yet, as few as 25 percent of them stated precisely that the reason for wishing to have hours remain unchanged was that they are presently meeting their course objectives. And 8.69 percent indicated a desire to decrease their clinical laboratory hours.

It is interesting to note in the belief items on guidance, that 10.32 percent of the faculty members see themselves in the nurse role instead of the teacher role in the clinical laboratory. Yet, in a corresponding belief item, only 4.34 percent stated that they saw themselves serving as a model of a nurse. Thus, we see that 5.98 percent perceive themselves as nurses in one situation and as teachers in another. This inconsistency in the perception of their role is intriguing. One wonders whether or not nurse faculty are really clear about their role.

Also, in the area of guidance, more than one-half of the sample (53.26 percent) stated that they believe the ratio of students to faculty could not be safely increased even if students in their course were to come to the clinical laboratory with an increased amount of knowledge about their activities. These figures are in contrast to the responses to the belief item on guidance, in which 99.45 percent stated that they believe that the learner should be guided to function independently. Higher ratios of students to faculty would seem to be consistent with independent action.

Three-fourths of the respondents (71.73 percent) indicated the belief that the central purpose of the clinical laboratory in nursing education is to provide an opportunity to apply theory to practice. More than one-fourth (25.54 percent) selected the mixture concept that dealt with the idea that students acquire knowledge through exposure to the real situation. Five respondents, or 2.71 percent, selected the worker concept that stated that students in a service profession learn by doing. These findings are in contrast to the tabulations on a preceding item in which 97.82 percent answered that they believe that students should experiment and discover courses of action in the clinical laboratory. Because experimentation involves the application of knowledge to practice, more consistent answers on these two questions were expected.

Whereas 86.41 percent of the respondents believe that the clinical laboratory activities of students in their course develop their creative abilities, 76.63 percent stated that nursing students are less creative than they could be. Reasons given by respondents for a lack of creativity by nursing students are disinterest in learning, grade consciousness, judgmental attitudes of faculty, rigid environment in clinical laboratory, and teachers' lack of knowledge of how to stimulate creativity.

Summary of Faculty Responses on Clinical Laboratory Activities

The percentage of responses that reflected the laboratory concept varied from element to element. Variability between items on the various components of the same element was also noted. The figures reflect the fact that the worker concept was least favored by the respondents. The greatest percentage of responses was spread between the laboratory concept and the mixture concept. Table A.1 presents the mean percentage of responses to the laboratory, mixture, and worker concepts on each essential element. Figure A.1 presents a graphic view of similar data.

TABLE A.1. Mean Percentage of Responses to Laboratory, Mixture, and Worker Concepts on Each Essential Element

| | Mean Percentage of Responses | | | |
Element	L	M	W	No Response
1. Critical thinking	72.46	13.67	13.22	0.63
2. Team concept	65.34	7.88	25.40	1.35
3. Professional judgment	64.40	9.91	24.04	1.62
4. Creativity	63.97	18.39	16.68	0.93
5. Experimentation	53.15	36.08	9.34	1.41
6. Skill learning	47.93	20.10	30.97	0.97
7. Guidance	46.91	50.63	1.71	0.75
8. Integrative activities	44.15	24.85	30.43	0.54
9. Patient contact	41.57	51.76	5.84	0.80
10. Objectives	41.03	39.80	17.52	1.63
11. Problem solving	40.62	47.27	10.99	1.08
12. Transfer of knowledge	34.23	46.55	17.38	1.81
13. Observation	27.71	32.06	38.70	1.17
14. Individuation	27.61	41.93	27.47	2.98

There is some overlap between the components of the essential elements. For example, prior knowledge is necessary for both expermentation and critical thinking. Questions on the use of prior knowledge were included on both elements and findings reported for each. Some apparent repetition also served as a source of cross-tabulation. Differences were noted among such responses.

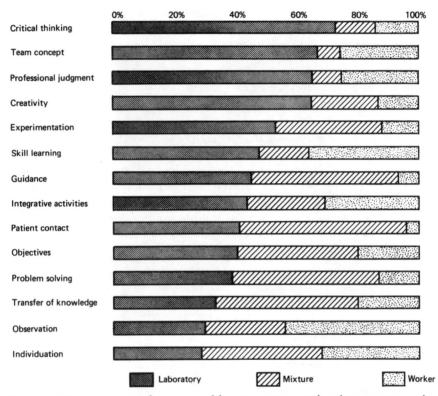

Figure A.1 Mean percentage of responses to laboratory, mixture, and worker concept on each essential element in order of predominance of the laboratory choices.

The percentage of laboratory concept responses to the teacher responsibility-centered elements was found to be lower than to most of the learner-centered elements. Three of these four elements ranked among the lowest of all the elements in the laboratory concept.

The percentage of the laboratory concept responses to the learner-centered elements varied from a low of 27.71 percent on observation to a high of 72.46 percent on critical thinking. The other-centered element, or team concept element, ranked second highest in percentage of responses to the laboratory concept.

Similarities and Differences Between Beliefs and Actions of Faculty

Cross-tabulations were done between the responses on selected belief items and do items. The essential elements selected for these cross-tabulations were those elements for which items had been constructed in both the belief and do parts of the instrument.

For the most part, examination of the results of the cross-tabulations between the belief and do items reveals that a generally low percentage of the respondents who express a belief in the laboratory concept actually practice this concept in their clinical teaching. In the majority of the situations analyzed, fewer than 50 percent of the respondents who stated that they believed in the laboratory concept selected the laboratory option on a do item on the same element. In a few situations a moderate percentage (50 to 60 percent) of the respondents who selected the laboratory concept on a belief item also selected the laboratory concept on a corresponding do item.

The element of professional judgment was the only element in which the cross-tabulations revealed consistently high agreement between the belief and do items. In three instances tabulated, more than 60 percent of the respondents expressed a belief in the laboratory concept and also indicated that they practice this concept in their teaching. It is interesting to note that professional judgment also ranked third highest among the other elements on the number of responses made to the laboratory concept option.

Other elements that ranked high on the selection of the laboratory concept response showed only low to moderate agreement between the belief and do items. On the element of critical thinking, which ranked first on laboratory responses, only one-third to two-thirds of those who stated a belief in the element indicated that they practice it. A single cross-tabulation was done on the skill-learning element, which ranked sixth highest on laboratory responses. Only one respondent checked the laboratory concept on both items. This person was the sole respondent who not only stated that laboratory sessions are better scheduled for a short period of time, but more frequently, and actually extended the idea to her course. The greater preponderance of responses on both items was on the worker concept.

A look at all of the cross-tabulations that involved two Yes-No items revealed that the greatest percentage of those respondents who did not select the laboratory concept on both items tended to select the laboratory concept on the belief item and not on the do item. In other words, the greater percentage of responses, in most of these instances, was in the cell corresponding to an expressed belief in the laboratory concept and an absence of evidence of the practice of this concept. This type of finding indicates an ineffective application of knowledge or belief to practice.

The following tendencies were noted on cross-tabulations that involved items in which one or both of them had a laboratory mixture-worker option. First, when the percentage of responses was low on both the belief and practice of the laboratory concept, the percentage of responses tended to be high on the belief of the laboratory concept and the practice of the mixture concept. This finding was true on the majority of the items for which cross-tabulations were done. Second, the tendency to select the option on the belief in the laboratory concept and the practice of the worker concept was noted in very few instances. However, on two elements this latter tendency was noted. On the elements of critical thinking and creativity, the tendency for those who stated a belief in these elements was to select the worker concept over the mixture concept. In one instance, on critical thinking, a larger percentage selected the worker concept than either the laboratory or mixture concept. In these specific areas the faculty responses showed that the worker concept was, in fact, operating in clinical laboratory activities.

Because observation ranked so low on the percentage of responses to the laboratory concept, it is interesting to note the findings of the cross-tabulations on this element. In one instance, there is a nearly even distribution of responses among the three concepts on the part of those who expressed a belief in the element. The worker concept, however, had the highest percentage of responses. In a second comparison, those who expressed the belief in observation in the clinical laboratory were distributed among the mixture concept and worker concept responses on the do item. There was only one exception. One respondent selected the laboratory concept on the do item. The findings seem to indicate confusion on the part of respondents as to how to implement the laboratory concept in regard to observation. Practice by teachers in the clinical laboratory is largely oriented to the worker or mixture concept on this element.

Another view of the findings is suggested as a result of the cross-tabulation of the belief and do items. Where there are both belief and practice of the laboratory concept on an element, there is no gap between theory and practice. Where there is an expressed belief in an element, but no practice evident, the gap is on the do side. Ineffective use is suggested. Where no belief is expressed and practice is evident, the gap is on the belief side and suggests that chance or ignorance is operating. Where there is agreement, but on the negative side, that is, no belief expressed and no practice of the laboratory concept evident, ignorance or obsolescence may be operating.

Relationship Between Characteristics of the Respondents and Their Responses

General findings reveal that the personal and professional characteristics of the respondents had very little effect on their responses. The similarity in the percentage of responses on each variable to each of the three concepts was astounding. In each of the variables or characteristics considered, a similar proportion of respondents selected the laboratory concept, the mixture concept, and the worker concept. Also, in each category of each variable, a larger number selected the laboratory concept, a smaller number selected the mixture concept, and still fewer selected the worker concept. The picture was surprisingly similar in each category and for each variable.

In each of the four age categories approximately one-half of the respondents in that category selected the laboratory concept. A lower percentage of respondents selected the mixture concept; a still lower percentage selected the worker concept. The proportionate percentages of responses in each category, to each of the three concepts, were nearly equal.

Approximately one-half of the respondents who graduated from a diploma school of nursing and one-half of those who graduated from a baccalaureate school of nursing selected the laboratory concept option. There was very little difference among the responses to the other two concepts.

A similar picture is presented in regard to the type of graduate education that the respondents had received. About one-half of those who had content in teaching on the graduate level selected the laboratory concept. The same is true of those who did not have content in teaching in their graduate program. The picture is only slightly different when practice in teaching on the graduate level is considered. Fifty-one percent of the respondents who had practice teaching in graduate school selected the laboratory concept; 47 percent of those who did not have practice teaching selected the laboratory concept.

The same distribution of responses on all three concepts occurred among the group that holds the associate degree and the group that holds the doctoral degree. Forty percent of those who hold the baccalaureate degree selected the laboratory concept, while 50 percent of those who hold the master's degree selected the laboratory concept. Those who hold the master's degree also were the group who least favored the worker concept.

On each of the other characteristics, such as area of specialization, year of graduation from basic program, and faculty rank, very little difference in response was noted.

Summary of the Findings

The findings in general revealed that although the great majority of the respondents expressed a belief in the essential elements specified, a much smaller percentage stated that they use the laboratory concept of these elements in clinical laboratory activities. In some specific situations the laboratory concept appears to be operating in a high percentage of the responses, such as on some items on guidance and creativity.

An examination of the collective response to each of the elements reveals that the laboratory concept was selected in approximately one-half of the responses. The other half of the responses contained a combination of the mixture concept and the worker concept. The worker concept was the least favored response.

Cross-tabulations between the belief and do items revealed that a generally low percentage of the respondents who express a belief in the laboratory concept actually practice this concept in their clinical teaching. In many instances a fairly large percentage of those who stated a belief in the laboratory concept of an element selected the mixture concept on a do item corresponding to that element. In a few instances a large number of respondents selected the belief item and the worker concept, such as on items on skill learning and observation.

In a consideration of the relationship between the personal and professional characteristics of the respondents and their responses, it was discovered that the characteristics considered had very little, if any, effect on the way they responded. Approximately the same percentage of responses was tabulated for each of the three concepts on each of the categories of characteristics.

Conclusions

The following conclusions regarding the clinical laboratory in baccalaureate nursing education were reached.

1. *The laboratory concept is used by a low to moderate percentage of faculty members in clinical laboratory activities in baccalaureate education in nursing.* Although the percentage of laboratory concept responses was relatively high on the elements of critical thinking, team concept, professional judgment, and creativity; in the remaining elements the percentage was surprisingly low. The contrast between the high percentage of responses expressing a belief in the elements and the low percentage of responses on the items involving practice of the elements in clinical laboratory is striking. However, the literature on the clinical laboratory in nursing shows that this conclusion was not entirely unexpected.

2. *There appears to be a trend away from the use of the worker concept by faculty members in clinical laboratory activities in baccalaureate education in nursing.* The worker concept was the least favored response in the majority of the items. Although the worker concept was selected rather infrequently and the laboratory concept was not in evidence as much as would be desired, the mixture concept was very much in evidence. The laboratory concept was selected in approximately half the responses. The mixture concept was selected in approximately one-third of the responses, while the worker concept was selected in approximately one-fourth of the responses. However, great variation was noted among the separate ele-

ments. In the teacher responsibility-centered elements, the mixture concept consistently received the highest percentage of the responses. Although there was more variability among the learner-centered elements, the mixture concept received a higher percentage of the responses in five of the nine elements.

Thus it can be concluded that baccalaureate nursing education appears to be moving away from the worker concept approach to clinical laboratory activities, yet it has not yet become sophisticated enough to move completely into the educationally oriented laboratory concept. The movement is currently caught largely in the mixture concept, which can be visualized as a compromise or cross section between the laboratory concept and the worker concept. However, the contamination of the old worker concept, although sometimes hidden, is still very much in evidence.

3. *Clinical laboratory activities provided for students were found to be very much oriented to caring for patients.* The greatest frequency of responses often occurred on the option that involved *caring*. The data inferred that a high percentage of clinical laboratory activities involved the student giving care to patients. It was in these situations that the mixture concept often received the highest percentage of the responses. Opportunity for the student to develop skill in each of the learner-centered elements was expected to be provided through activities involving the student giving direct care to patients. For example, the student is expected to learn to make observations while rendering care to patients. It would seem that the respondents were unable to discriminate between caring for patients and learning how to care for patients.

Also, the data implied that the student's practice in the clinical laboratory is expected to proceed without error. Whereas error that could be critical to a patient's well-being must be avoided by proper preparation for clinical laboratory activities, learners are expected to profit from some error. Teachers should not only expect errors, but they should not punish students for errors. Teachers should also expect, however, that students correct their own errors.

This overconcern on the part of the faculty for the care of patients is intriguing, especially in view of the fact that the vast majority of them stated that they see themselves as teachers, not nurses. Despite what these teachers say, their teaching strategies still demonstrate that the question raised by Burns[2] is still very much with us. The question is whether faculty in these programs are nurses who happen to be teachers or teachers who happen to be nurses. They apparently verbalize what they know they should believe and then proceed to behave otherwise.

Although patient contact is essential to clinical laboratory activities, the type of patient contact provided for students by the respondents in this study was not always educationally oriented. The responses indicated that learners were often tied to the responsibilities of patient care. The responsibility for care and the responsibility for service cannot be satisfied simultaneously. One must often yield to the other.

4. *Much inconsistency was evidenced between the belief and action on the part of participants in the study.* The data showed a lack of consistency between the verbalizations and the behavior of the respondents. Many respondents expressed a belief in the laboratory concept. Few respondents evidenced practice of the essential elements of this concept in the clinical laboratory. Faculty members had a wide variety of opinions and ideas about what clinical laboratory activities should be and how they should be provided and guided. This variation was evidenced in responses to the do items.

The determination of reasons for this finding was not within the scope of this study, but this contrast in responses suggests uncertainty. The uncertainty seems to be centered on how faculty beliefs can be realized in practice. Perhaps a lack of knowledge or the lack of ability to apply theory to practice in teaching is at the root of the problem. Further study would be indicated.

5. *Nurse faculty members provide much individual time and attention to students.* The highest percentage of laboratory concept responses occurred on a number of elements in situations that involved interaction between student and teacher. By and large, faculty discuss clinical laboratory activities with individual students and spend much time with each of them in the clinical laboratory. This conclusion in and of itself might seem to be a positive one. Yet, in view of the fact that the laboratory concept options on the individuation element drew the smallest number of responses, a question is raised as to the type and quality of guidance given to students.

Is it actually guidance that is being rendered, or is it elbow supervision? Is it really guidance, or is it hovering that tends to stifle the imagination and independence of the student? Nurse faculty tend to be overly guidance oriented. Or perhaps it would be more accurate to say that they are overly supervision oriented. Another question that is raised is whether the reason for this tendency is *primarily* motivated by concern for the learning of the student or for the care of the patient. The data suggest that guidance is oriented to the prevention of errors by the student.

6. *The responses to the laboratory concept were not affected by the various characteristics of the respondents.* Differences among the type of responses made by these faculty members that could be attributed to age or type of education were essentially nonexistent. Newer teaching strategies or supposedly updated curricula, of which the younger age group were a product, had no noticeable effect on their responses. There were essentially no differences in the way diploma school graduates and baccalaureate graduates responded. There was only a slightly higher percentage of responses to the laboratory concept by those who had a practicum in teaching in their gradu-

ate program as opposed to those who did not. In fact, approximately the same percentage of responses was tabulated for each of the three concepts on each of the categories of characteristics.

Question is raised as to whether or not the respondents actually do what they say they do. Through the use of a questionnaire, a researcher finds out what a respondent says he does but not, in effect, what he does. The respondents often know what they should do, and this influences how they respond. The possibility exists that data collected by direct observation of faculty may yield different findings.

Some of the questions in the instrument circumvented this problem better than others. Where a direct question about what was actually being done was asked, a low percentage of respondents answered according to the laboratory concept. When a hypothetical situation was used as a point of reference, a higher percentage of respondents tended to select the laboratory concept. In the latter situation it was possible for the respondent to determine the principle that was being tested for and answer according to the desirable response. If this phenomenon was indeed operating, it suggests that faculty know the correct answer, but cannot, will not, or do not believe in actuating it in their clinical teaching.

Suggestions for Future Research

This study surveyed the clinical laboratory activities in selected baccalaureate programs in nursing. Further studies might be conducted to expand and validate these findings. Others might also test the results of changes that could be tried as an outcome of the findings of this research.

For example, a replication of this study could be done in other geographic regions to compare findings. Direct observations of the behavior of faculty and students in the clinical laboratory could be made to compare findings with the responses to a questionnaire. These observations could be based on the essential elements. Also, experimental studies could be performed in a manner designed to test the effectiveness of teaching strategies in the clinical laboratory specifically introduced to utilize the laboratory concept in relation to one or more of the essential elements.

Notes

1. Kluckhohn, F., & Strodtbeck, F. *Variations in Value Orientations.* New York: Row, Peterson and Company, 1961, p. 437.
2. Burns, M. E. *Faculty opinions on their academic responsibilities in baccalaureate nursing programs.* Unpublished doctoral dissertation, Teachers College, Columbia University, 1969, p. 133.

Index

199